The Brain Atlas

*A Visual Guide to the Human
Central Nervous System*

The Brain Atlas

A Visual Guide to the Human Central Nervous System

Joseph Hanaway, M.D.
Clinical Assistant Professor of Neurology
Washington University School of Medicine
Attending Neurologist
St. Mary's Health Center
St. Louis, Missouri

Thomas A. Woolsey, M.D.
George H. and Ethel R. Bishop Scholar in Neuroscience
Professor of Neurology and Neurological Surgery,
of Anatomy and Neurobiology, and of Cell Biology and Physiology
Washington University School of Medicine
St. Louis, Missouri

Mokhtar H. Gado, M.D.
Professor of Radiology
Mallinckrodt Institute of Radiology
Washington University School of Medicine
St. Louis, Missouri

Melville P. Roberts, Jr., M.D.
William Beecher Scoville Professor of Neurosurgery
University of Connecticut School of Medicine
Farmington, Connecticut
Senior Attending Neurosurgeon
Hartford Hospital
Hartford, Connecticut

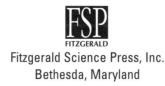

Fitzgerald Science Press, Inc.
Bethesda, Maryland

Fitzgerald Science Press, Inc.
Editorial Offices
Bethesda, Maryland
(301) 229–1134
fitzscipress@msn.com

Fitzgerald Science Press, Inc.
Orders and Fulfillment:
P.O. Box 605
Herndon, VA 20172
(800) 869–4409
(703) 661–1577
Fax (703) 661–1501

Library of Congress Cataloging-in-Publication Data
The brain atlas: a visual guide to the human central
nervous system/Joseph Hanaway...[et al.].
      p.   cm.
   Includes bibliographical references and index.
   ISBN 1-891786-05-9 (pbk.). –ISBN 1-891786-06-7 (hardcover)
   1. Brain–Anatomy–Atlases. 2. Central nervous system–
Anatomy–Atlases. I. Hanaway, Joseph, 1933- .
   [DNLM: 1. Brain–anatomy & histology atlases. 2. Central Nervous
System–anatomy & histology atlases. WL 17 B814 1998]
QM455.B633 1998
611'.0022'2–dc21
DNLM/DLC
for Library of Congress   98-20351
                          CIP

The paperback edition of this work (ISBN: 1 891786-05-9) is
distributed outside the USA and Canada exclusively by
Oxford University Press.
Address orders and inquiries to:
  OUP Distribution Services
  Saxon Way West
  Corby Northants NN18 9ES
  Tel: +44 (0) 1536 741519

98 99 00 01 02—10 9 8 7 6 5 4 3 2

The publisher dedicates this work to the memory of
Kevin M. Doyle and David S. McEttrick.

Dedicated to

Clinton N. Woolsey

Jerzy E. Rose

David Bodian

Francis MacNaughton

Andrew Rasmussen

James W. Bull

George du Boulay

William Beecher Scoville

Table of Contents

2. Axial Sections

3. Sagittal Sections

Part IV. Histological Sections

1. Spinal Cord

2. Brain Stem and Cerebellum

3. Basal Ganglia and Thalamus

4. Hypothalamus, Basal Forebrain, and Hippocampus

Part V. Pathways

Index

Preface

The Decade of the Brain (1990–2000) has seen an exciting systematic worldwide push to greater understanding of brain function in health and disease. From basic neurobiology to human brain mapping, a primary aim now is to unravel how the human brain works. The explosion of new knowledge and new concepts is breathtaking. Opportunities are expanding rapidly for relating both newer findings and older classical knowledge to real images of the living human brain. For the first time, it is possible to observe the detailed structure of a person's brain as that individual matures, ages, suffers from disease, and recovers. A fundamental understanding of the structural organization of the central nervous system is essential to comprehend this new information.

The growing interest in brain function and the increased incidence of diseases affecting the brain in a maturing population have not been matched by the time allotted to teach and to study the structure of the human nervous system. Indeed, in many medical schools and universities, scheduled time for direct interaction between students and professors has been sharply curtailed. Yet clinicians and researchers alike are compelled to be ever more familiar with the actual structure of the brain and spinal cord as they are now routinely seen in wonderful detail by magnetic resonance imaging (MRI) in living persons. Thus, there is a need for a focused atlas of brain structure to provide a visual guide for teachers, students, and the other health care workers who have less scheduled time in which to master the subject.

The Brain Atlas: A Visual Guide to the Human Central Nervous System meets this need. It is built on the original pictures of brain sections first published by two of us in the *Atlas of the Human Brain in Section* (Roberts et al., 1987), using a labeling style that has proven exceptionally effective for learning. *The Brain Atlas: A Visual Guide to the Human Central Nervous System* adds substantially to the superb pictures of brain slices and sections from the earlier work:

• new dissections demonstrate the major features of the human brain, including the blood vessels;

• high-quality MRI scans are matched directly to the brain slices to guide direct correlations in the clinic;

• selected neuroradiological images are arranged to permit easy comparison with pictures of the brain and its arteries;

• areas of the brain supplied by each blood vessel are mapped on the dissections, slices, and selected sections; and

• histological sections through the hypothalamus, thalamus, and forebrain provide excellent detail of these regions.

Innovative diagrams of the principal neuronal pathways that directly use the images of specimens, slices, and sections depicted in the plates are made possible by computers. Pathway diagrams have been rendered to convey the three-dimensional character of the principal connections of the brain in living persons. The labeling with leaders and numbers facilitates group teaching and self-testing. The book has been designed in an uncluttered style to permit rapid location of plates by brain region or topic.

Today most of the major structures of the brain can be seen in living subjects by MRI and other techniques. These techniques are improving daily; reports of new discoveries about the brain also appear with increasing frequency. In *The Brain Atlas: A Visual Guide to the Human Central Nervous System,* we have provided enough detail to make it a useful reference and course adjunct for medical and other health care students, but also for neuropathologists; radiologists; residents in neurology, neurosurgery, and psychiatry; selected heath care personnel; psychologists; cognitive scientists; and interested laypersons.

Acknowledgments

This book could not have been made without the excellent assistance of the following persons: James Nelson, M.D., and Adrianne Noe, Ph.D., for access to and assistance with the Yakovlev-Haleem slide collection in the National Museum of Health and Medicine (a Division of the Armed Forces Institute of Pathology); Martin M. Henegar, M.D., for some of the dissections; S. Thomas Carmichael, M.D., Ph. D., and Arthur D. Loewy, Ph.D., for updates on some of the connections; J. Gayle King for help with the cadaveric specimens; Walter Clermont for photography of brain specimens; and Thomas Murry of the Mallinckrodt Institute of Radiology for photography of radiological images. Brain icons are after original sketches by Melville P. Roberts, Jr., M.D. Special thanks to Mike Demaray and J/B Woolsey Associates for illustration, layout, and pre-production. Kathy Diekmann facilitated the meetings of authors and movement of materials among all parties. We thank Drs. Arthur Loewy and Allan Siegel and many of our colleagues for their comments prior to this revised printing. Support from the Spastic Paralysis Foundation of the Illinois—Eastern Iowa District of Kiwanis International to Dr. Woolsey is gratefully acknowledged. Cindy Woolsey and Nancy Hanaway are tolerant true heroines.

The Brain Atlas

*A Visual Guide to the Human
Central Nervous System*

Background Information

Background Information

Overview

The Layout of the Book

The Brain Atlas: A Visual Guide to the Human Central Nervous System is arranged in five parts:

Part I contains selected background information, tips for using the book, descriptions of methods, and valuable general references.

Part II illustrates the three-dimensional appearance of the brain (life-size). It is our experience that scientists and caregivers alike need constantly to be reminded that the brain and its blood vessels in the head of a living patient or experimental subject are not isolated, as in an anatomical specimen, but are in a context, as seen in MRIs. Accordingly—and unique to *The Brain Atlas: A Visual Guide to the Human Central Nervous System*—the plates in Part II are grouped on facing pages to show the dissected brain with and without blood vessels and with the major arterial territories. Selected radiograms are integrated as groups of plates to correlate with these vessels in the living.

Part III presents the beautiful pictures of brain slices (again life-size) that were the outstanding feature of the *Atlas of the Human Brain in Section* by Roberts et al. (1987). These are the core of *The Brain Atlas: A Visual Guide to the Human Central Nervous System*. The sections proceed systematically through the brain in the three cardinal planes. A major new feature of *The Brain Atlas: A Visual Guide to the Human Central Nervous System* is the addition of plates facing each slice showing either a carefully matched MRI or the outline of the territories of the main arteries supplying regions in the slice.

Part IV illustrates low-power microscopic organization of the brain. To the plates of myelin-stained sections of the brain stem and spinal cord from the Roberts atlas, *The The Brain Atlas: A Visual Guide to the Human Central Nervous System* adds sections through the cerebellum, basal ganglia, thalamus, hypothalamus, hippocampus, and basal forebrain. Plates showing the sections through the cerebellum, basal ganglia, spinal cord, and the brain stem also illustrate the territories of the principal arteries supplying them.

Part V combines selected images from Parts II, III, and IV into novel illustrations of the main neural pathways in the human brain. Computer-based illustration permitted the authors to direct the artist's "pen" precisely. Students and working health care personnel can move easily back and forth between a pathway's depiction in Part V to the plates used to compose it in Parts II, III, and IV to clarify structure, neighbor relationships, and blood supply. A short synopsis describes the function and connections of each pathway.

Terminology

Correct names and terms for structures in the brain are essential for clear communication, and they are constantly changing as more is learned about the brain. Preference for terminologies based on the spoken language of faculty and students is a worldwide trend. This has been recognized by the International Federation of Associations of Anatomists (IFAA). The latest nomenclature adopted by the IFAA's Federative Committee on Anatomical Terminology (FCAT) is used in *The Brain Atlas: A Visual Guide to the Human Central Nervous System*. The terminology in *The Brain Atlas: A Visual Guide to the Human Central Nervous System* is largely English (*part* for *pars*) or taken from the older Latin, Greek, and Egyptian terms of anatomy and medicine that are now part of the English language (substantia nigra, thalamus). However, a complete conversion to FCAT terms is premature in many instances, and in such instances, the term commonly used is followed by the FCAT term equivalent in parentheses, for example, gyrus rectus (straight gyrus). Commonly used synonyms and eponyms also are indicated in parentheses: corticospinal (pyramidal) tract; basal vein (basal vein of *Rosenthal*).

For structures composed of several parts, the principal structure is followed by the specific part(s), separated by a comma: hippocampus, CA3, pyramidal layer; thalamus, centromedian nucleus (CM); fourth ventricle (IV), median aperture (foramen of *Magendie*). Terms for nuclei in the thalamus include an abbreviation in parentheses: centromedian nucleus (CM); ventral posteromedial nucleus (VPMm), medial part; thalamus, pulvinar (Pul). Cranial nerves (CN) and associated structures are numbered with capital Roman numerals: vagal (CN X) trigone; trigeminal nerve (CN V); abducent nucleus (CN VI). The third and fourth ventricles are indicated with capital Roman numerals: fourth ventricle (IV), median aperture (foramen of *Magendie*).

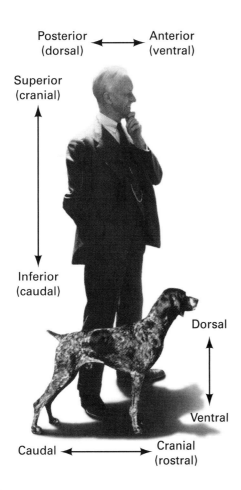

Figure 1. Terms of comparison applied to a human and a quadruped.

Adjectives describing anatomical relations are well discussed in textbooks of anatomy. In *The Brain Atlas: A Visual Guide to the Human Central Nervous System,* FCAT adjectives are used, but commonly used synonyms of relation are included in parentheses: posterior (dorsal) horn; anterior (ventral) cochlear nucleus (CN VIII). The interchangeable use of some terms of comparison as related to humans and quadrupeds in the literature and in medicine can be confusing (Figure 1). In the dog, the axis of the forebrain is the same as the axis of the spinal cord, while in the human, the axis of the forebrain is at nearly 90° to the axis of the spinal cord. Structures within the human forebrain that are nearer the back of the head (occiput) are posterior with respect to the principal body axis, for example, the occipital (posterior) horn of the lateral ventricle. Whereas in dogs, a structure in the same relative position will be nearer the tail (caudal) than to the back (dorsal), and so forth. In the FCAT, *pontine reticular formation (superior part)* is preferred over the traditional

usage, *rostral reticular formation.* The lists give the preferred term with the synonym in parentheses: anterior (ventral) horn; posterior (dorsal) spinocerebellar tract. In some instances, the use of quadruped relations, unfortunately, cannot be avoided: *dorsal* supraoptic commissure; thalamus, latero*dorsal* nucleus (LD) – not *superior.*

Labeling

The labeling system in *The Brain Atlas: A Visual Guide to the Human Central Nervous System* was devised after considering and testing all available formats. Numbers, generally arranged in clockwise order, allow the reader to locate a structure immediately without an extensive search to find a specific symbol or term against the background of a structure. A systematic numbering code (e.g., caudate nucleus, head = 23) has been avoided on purpose so that the lists of terms for each plate can be covered and the numbers used for self-testing (Figure 2). Where several plates in a group are related, as on facing pages, black type is used for structures on the first figure in the group (to the left) and the same structures on other figures in the group. Red type is used for structures that are first identified on the subsequent figures in the group.

Leaders are used so that numbers can be arranged in order for rapid identification of structures. The structures are much better seen when leaders are used than when

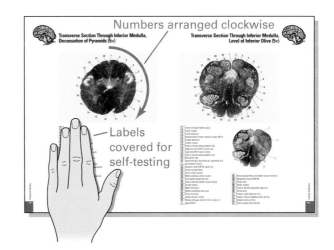

Figure 2. Structures are identified by leaders which are numbered clockwise from 12 o'clock. Each number has a term spelled out in the list which can be covered for self-testing.

labels are placed directly on the images (see *Brodmann*'s areas in Figure 6). Leaders permit greater precision, particularly for identification of smaller features. Because of the large number of items in each plate, it is impractical to label all of them on every section. Larger structures (e.g., caudate nucleus, lateral ventricle) that appear in adjacent sections have been labeled on alternate plates or less frequently. Students are encouraged to try to identify unlabeled structures as a self-testing exercise.

Pathways and Pathway Diagrams

Neural pathways are depicted with "stacks" of selected images (specimens, slices, and histological sections) in a three-quarter view as if seen from the left front. This perspective was chosen because it gives a sense of the three dimensions not appreciated in the elegant illustration style developed by Rasmussen (1932) that has been so widely imitated. To obtain these views, images of the sections were rotated and "extruded" to create a sense of true perspective. They are aligned with respect to the central canal of the spinal cord and closed medulla, the median longitudinal fissure of the fourth ventricle, and the cerebral aqueduct. Section images were adjusted so that relative sizes are preserved—sacral cord < cervical cord < medulla < isthmus < pons < thalamus—but true sizes vary because, for instance, the section of sacral cord would be too small for gray and white matter to be resolved if it were reproduced at the same magnification as a midbrain section. The pathways shown are simplified from the highly detailed information now available from humans and primates (e.g., Paxinos, 1990). In some cases, such as the hypothalamospinal tract, we have transposed data from nonprimates that is consistent with clinical observation in humans, for example, lateral medullary syndrome. A short synopsis accompanies each pathway diagram, summarizing its function(s) and the structures connected.

Brain Basics

Cerebrospinal Fluid, Ventricles, Choroid Plexus, and Subarachnoid Space. The lumen of the neural tube persists in the spinal cord and closed medulla as the central canal; in the rest of the brain, it expands into the ventricular system. The choroid plexus, a specialized secretory epithelium found in each ventricle (Figure 3), actively generates ≈700 cc cerebrospinal fluid a day. The brain and spinal cord are filled and bathed by ≈150 cc cerebrospinal fluid that circulates from and fills the ventricles, the central canal, and the subarachnoid space between the pia on the brain surface and the arachnoidal membrane just under the dura. Widened regions of the subarachnoid space are called cisterns.

The Central Nervous System. The central nervous system (CNS) is protected in the cranial cavity of the skull and in the spinal canal formed by the neural arches. The adult brain weighs between 1250 and 1450 g and occupies ≈1400 cc. The adult spinal cord is approximately 50 cm long and occupies ≈150 cc. Both arise in early development from a single tube, the neural tube, which greatly expands in the front end of the embryo to form the main three divisions of the brain, two of which later differentiate into two additional divisions each (Figure 4). The adult brain therefore consists of the telencephalon, which includes the cerebral cortex, basal ganglia, and olfactory bulbs; the diencephalon, which includes the thalamus, hypothalamus, and habenula (epithalamus); the mesencephalon or midbrain, which includes structures around the cerebral aqueduct, the superior and inferior colliculi, and the cerebral peduncles; the metencephalon, which includes the pons and cerebellum; and the myelencephalon ("spinal cord-like"), which includes the open and closed medulla.

Spine, Spinal Cord, and Spinal Roots. The relationships of the spinal column, spinal roots, and spinal cord deserve comment. The spinal column consists of 33 vertebrae: 7 vertebrae in the neck (cervical, C1-C7), 12 in the thorax (T1-T12), 5 in the abdomen (lumbar, L1-L5), 5 in the pelvis (sacral, S1-S5), and 4 in the diminutive "tail" (coccygeal, Co1-Co4). The spinal cord lies within the bony spinal canal of the spinal column and consists of 31 segments (8 cervical, 12 thoracic, 5 lumbar, 5 sacral, and 1 coccygeal), each giving rise to a pair of spinal nerves (e.g., C1, T1, L1, S1, Co1) (Figure 5). Each pair of spinal nerves exits the bony spinal canal between two adjacent vertebrae, except superiorly where the first pair exits between the skull and C1. Each cervical root is therefore numbered by the vertebra *below* its exit. The last cervical nerve, C8, exits between vertebrae C7 and T1. Below C8, each spinal nerve, including T1, has the same number as the vertebra

1	Central sulcus (fissure of *Rolando*)
2	Choroid plexus of lateral ventricle
3	Lateral sulcus (*Sylvian* fissure)
4	Lateral ventricle, trigone (atrium)
5	Lateral ventricle, occipital (posterior) horn
6	Lateral ventricle, temporal (inferior) horn
7	Fourth ventricle (IV)
8	Cerebellum, hemisphere
9	Choroid plexus of fourth ventricle (IV)
10	Fourth ventricle (IV), median aperture (foramen of *Magendie*)
11	Medulla oblongata
12	Fourth ventricle (IV), lateral aperture (foramen of *Luschka*)
13	Pons
14	Cerebral aqueduct (aqueduct of *Sylvius*)
15	Choroid plexus of lateral ventricle, temporal (inferior) horn
16	Frontal pole
17	Lateral ventricle, frontal (anterior) horn
18	Interventricular foramen (foramen of *Monro*)
19	Third ventricle (III)
20	Lateral ventricle, body
21	Superior sagittal sinus
22	Interthalamic adhesion (massa intermedia)
23	Straight sinus
24	Occipital pole
25	Cerebellum, vermis
26	Midbrain
27	Pituitary gland
28	Septum pellucidum
29	Fornix
30	Corpus callosum
31	Arachnoid granulations

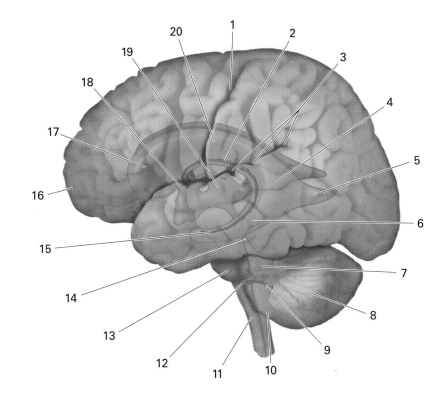

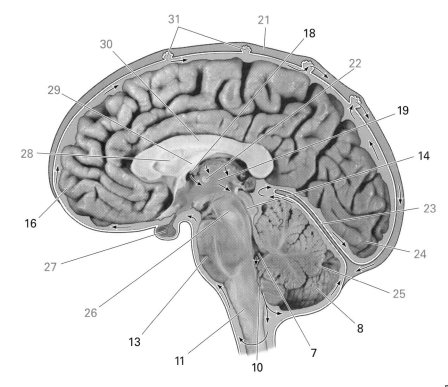

Figure 3. The location of the choroid plexus, which makes cerebrospinal fluid (CSF), is shown in the four brain ventricles (0.6x). CSF circulates through the ventricular system and over the brain, as shown by the arrows.

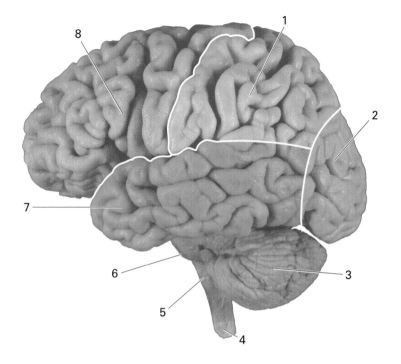

segments of the spinal cord (e.g., C1, T1, L1, S1, Co1). In the upper cervical region, a spinal cord segment lies at approximately the same level as the corresponding vertebra. Inferiorly, cord segments lie progressively at more superior levels than the corresponding vertebrae. The adult spinal cord ends at the level of the first lumbar vertebra (L1). The discrepancy between the cord and vertebral levels is due to differences in the growth of the spine and spinal cord. Nerve roots occupy the lumbar spinal canal below L1, where they constitute the cauda equina ("horse tail").

***Brodmann's* Areas in the Cerebral Cortex.** In *The Brain Atlas: A Visual Guide to the Human Central Nervous System* structures are identified by anatomical name at different levels of resolution. However, a system of numbering the different regions of the cerebral cortex is referred to in the book (Figure 6). In the past, these regions were defined by several investigators based on microscopic patterns of nerve cell bodies (cytoarchitectonics), of which the most widely

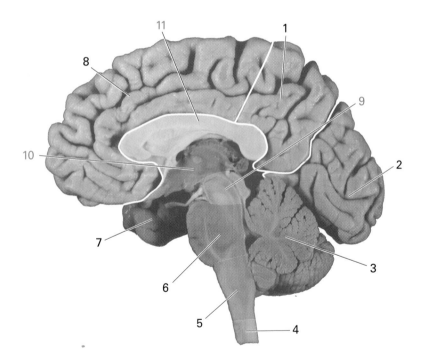

1	Parietal lobe
2	Occipital lobe
3	Cerebellum
4	Spinal cord
5	Medulla oblongata (myelencephalon)
6	Pons
7	Temporal lobe
8	Frontal lobe
9	Midbrain (Mesencephalon)
10	Hypothalamus, thalamus, habenula and pineal gland (diencephalon)
11	Corpus callosum, anterior commissure, fornix and septum pellucidum

1, 2, 7, 8, and 11. Telencephalon (Cerebral hemisphere)
1, 2, 7, 8, 10, and 11. Prosencephalon (Forebrain)
3 and 6. Metencephalon
3, 5, and 6. Rhombencephalon (Hindbrain)

Figure 4. The principal divisions of the brain labeled in lateral and midsagittal views.

used is a system of numbers published by Korbinian Brodmann in 1909. To a first approximation, these divisions—*Brodmann*'s areas (indicated by circled numbers)—correspond with known patterns of connections and separable brain functions. They are used to identify particular parts of the cortical mantle that are sources and targets of neural pathways (see Part V of this book).

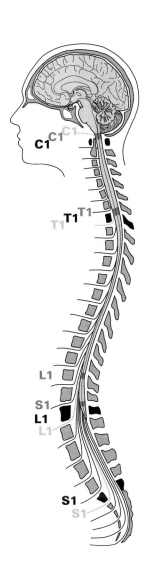

Figure 5. Levels of the spinal cord labeled red, spinal nerve roots yellow, and vertebral column black.

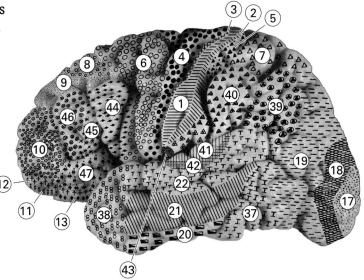

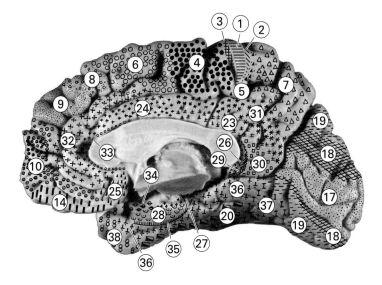

Figure 6. *Brodmann*'s system of numbers identify areas of the cerebral cortex by their microscopic structure. These numbers are used today, especially where they correspond to particular functions and connections.

How To Use This Book

The Brain Atlas: A Visual Guide to the Human Central Nervous System is not a textbook. Rather it is a reference that can be used as a student first begins to study the human brain and can be a source of clarification in the workaday world of medical practice and research. The parts of this book are arranged in sequence from the whole brain and its blood supply through the slices and histological sections to simple pathway diagrams. Each part is linked to the others, and once an overview is obtained, the parts should be used together to clarify a particular subject.

The plates are grouped for easy comparison; for instance, in Part II, different views of the brain with blood vessels are on facing pages (Figure 7). Smaller images show the brain territories supplied by the main vessels. These territories represent the main patterns of supply and do not indicate overlap in regions supplied or some of the variation normally encountered. Adjacent pages show radiological clinical studies of the blood vessels (Figure 8).

Part II can be used by novices (e.g., undergraduates interested in brain science and cognitive psychology) to familiarize themselves with the form of the brain, by health care students to refresh dissections, and by professionals to recall brain features. These images provide the big picture, and a three-dimensional sense of the life-size brain can be gotten after quick study. In the

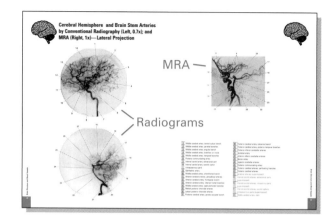

Figure 8. The arteries supplying the brain of a live person seen in radiological studies, which can be compared to the whole brain images.

radiological reading room, on a hospital floor, or in a doctor's office, these plates provide context for clinical images such as plain skull films, CT, or MRI.

Part III can be used directly to identify structures in brain slices studied in student laboratories and in neuropathology. In Part III, a brain slice may be grouped with an MRI that is matched to include virtually identical structures. Students are encouraged to carefully compare the plates on facing pages to place the principal image, which is always on the left-hand page, in a broader context, such as when considering MRI images from a patient or experimental subject. The adjacent pages show the territories supplied by vessels, which can be related to the MRI by flipping back and forth between them (Figure 9). Adjacent MRIs and vessel territories can be used to clarify questions arising from examination of cross-sectional images obtained in a clinical setting.

Part IV contains the sections of the core of the central nervous system. They can be used to identify structures, to place the neural pathways illustrated in Part V in detailed context, and to analyze symptom/sign complexes such as those found with the occlusion of a principal blood vessel supplying a region. Part IV can also be used to get finer definition of regions that can be appreciated generally on clinical images, such as tracts and nuclei of the brain stem or of the thalamus and parts of the hippocampus.

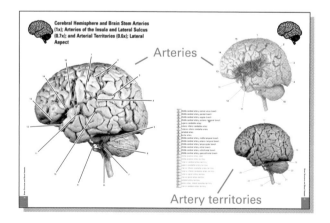

Figure 7. The arteries to the brain at the left dissected with their territories at the right.

Part V groups images of the specimens, slices, and sections together to illustrate the principal pathways in the brain. In studies of deficits arising from specific lesions to the brain, it is possible to use these diagrams in conjunction with images in Parts II–IV to clarify the involvement of the different pathways that give rise to the symptoms and signs in a particular clinical picture (Figure 10). The original sections can be found easily with the locator icons.

The Brain Atlas: A Visual Guide to the Human Central Nervous System has several features designed to assist in rapid location of pertinent figures and to permit easy navigation between the different parts of the book. The Parts are color coded: the colored page numbers and page edges make it easy to find a part of the book quick-

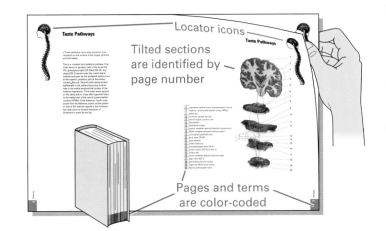

Figure 10. Brain pathways are drawn on tilted sections from other parts of the atlas. Color-coded sections of the book permit easy reference to different groups of plates. Locator diagrams in the upper corners of the pages can be flipped through to find a particular level or orientation through the brain.

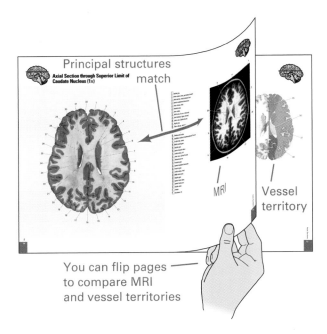

Figure 9. Selected brain slices are matched to MRIs. Adjacent brain slices are matched to outlines of the territories supplied by their arteries.

ly (Figure 10). Each group of plates has a locator icon in the upper outside corner of all pages. These help place the slice/section in context and will be useful in conjunction with locator images now common in clinical imaging. The corners can be flipped through quickly to find an approximate location for a section or a particular region (e.g., spinal cord vs. blood supply of the cerebellum).

Methods

Brain Specimens

Fixation. Brains were obtained from cadavers within 24 hours of death. Both common carotid arteries and vertebral arteries were exposed in the neck and clamped proximally. The jugular veins were transected. After flushing with normal NaCl, all vessels were perfused simultaneously with 16% paraformaldehyde in buffered normal saline from a reservoir 45 cm above the head. After 2 hours, when the neck was stiff, the head was removed and soft tissues of the skull dissected away. The skull was opened and the head stored for 3–4 weeks in 16% paraformaldehyde, which was changed weekly. The specimen depicted in most of the plates is from a 78-year-old woman who died from pneumonia. There was no clinical or pathological evidence of central nervous system disease or involvement.

Dissection. The skull was carefully removed to expose the dura and proximal internal carotid and vertebral arteries. Complete sets of photographs were taken as the dissections proceeded. The dura was opened and removed. The blood vessels were defined and then carefully removed by peeling the pia.

Photography. The specimens were photographed in black and white on large format (4x5) negatives. The negatives were digitized for labeling and coloring.

Brain Slices

Fixation. Brains were obtained at autopsy within 24 hours of death. As soon as the brain was removed, the vertebral and carotid arteries were each perfused with 50 ml of 40% formaldehyde. Brains were suspended by the basilar artery in 10% formalin for 2–4 weeks to complete fixation. The brain cut in the coronal plane is from a 22-year-old who died from a retroperitoneal hemangioendothelioma; that in the axial plane from a 58-year-old man who died from a renal adenocarcinoma; and that in the sagittal series from a 35-year-old woman who died from chronic renal failure. None showed clinical or pathological evidence for central nervous system disease or involvement.

Sectioning. Fixed brains were blocked for correct orientation using a brain knife (frontal lobes for the coronal plane and the vertex for the axial plane). They were sliced serially at 4 mm on a Hobart Model 410 rotary blade commercial meat slicer. The slices were stacked in order and separated by filter paper.

Staining. The brain slices were stained with a modified copper sulfate technique (Mulligan, 1931). The slices were washed in cold running tap water for 30 minutes. Each slice was then immersed in a pyrex baking dish for 6 minutes in 1.5 L of staining solution ($CuSO_4 \cdot 5H_2O$, 5 gm; phenol, 50 gm; 37.5% HCl, 1 ml in 1 L dH_2O) at 60°C. Each section was washed for 7 minutes in cold tap water and placed in 1.5 L of fresh 1.5% $K_4Fe(CN)_6 \cdot 3H_2O$ (30-60 sec until the gray matter turned red-brown. After washing for 6 minutes in running tap water, the sections can be stored in 10% formalin for several months without fading. Gray matter stains red-brown, while the white matter is unstained.

Photography. Sections were photographed through a green filter (Wratten #58 to enhance contrast) on large format (5x7) negatives with illuminated background. Final prints were made at ~1.2 X; these were digitized for labeling, shading, and rendering.

Histological Sections

Material. Sections shown in the Roberts et al., 1987 atlas were taken from normal brain stems and spinal cords. They were embedded in celloidin, cut at 40 μm, and stained by the Loyez method for myelin. Sections from the Yakovlev-Haleem Collection at the National Museum of Health and Medicine were chosen from many normal specimens to illustrate appropriate levels. The sections were embedded in celloidin and cut serially at 35–40 μm; alternate sections were stained by the Loyez method for myelin and cresyl violet for cell bodies (Nissl substance; e.g., Gabe, 1976).

Photography. The specimens were photographed in black and white on large format (4x5) negatives. The negatives were digitized for labeling and coloring.

Cerebral Angiography

Angiography is a technique for imaging blood vessels in

living persons. In conventional cerebral angiography, X-rays are used to make images when the blood vessels of the brain are filled by intravascular injection of radio-opaque contrast material (dye). Images are collected in rapid succession for approximately 10 seconds starting just before the dye is injected. Each frame includes an image of the head, skull, soft tissues, and contrast-filled blood vessels. The sequence of frames constitutes a *cerebral angiogram,* which is specified by the artery into which the contrast material is injected, for example, right carotid angiogram.

The contrast material circulates first into the cerebral arteries, the *arterial phase,* and collects several seconds later in the cerebral veins, the *venous phase.* The recording device for the images in this atlas was an image intensifier. Each frame was digitized on-line. A frame of the skull and soft tissues prior to entry of the contrast material was subtracted from subsequent frames to electronically "remove" the skull and demonstrate the blood vessels in isolation.

Cerebral angiograms are obtained in *views* or *projections* named by the path of X-rays in relation to the head. There are two basic views. In the *lateral view,* the X-rays cross from one side of the head to the other, perpendicular to the midsagittal plane (pages 26, 27, 29). In the *anteroposterior view* (pages 31–33), X-rays pass parallel to the midsagittal plane from the front to the back.

The lateral view of a carotid angiogram contains the blood vessels on both sides of a hemisphere as well as those within it deep to the surface, all superimposed. Likewise, in a vertebral angiogram that fills the basilar artery, the cerebellar arteries and the posterior cerebral arteries of both sides are superimposed in the lateral projection.

Magnetic Resonance Imaging

Magnetic resonance imaging (MRI) scanners contain a strong magnet, a radio frequency (RF) transmitter, a receiver (antenna), and a computer for processing the received signal. In strong magnetic fields, nuclei of hydrogen atoms, acting as little magnets, align in relation to the direction of the magnetic field attempting to reach a state of equilibrium (net magnetization). Hydrogen atoms within the magnetic field absorb the energy of a matched RF pulse, resulting in perturbation of their alignment. As they return to their magnetic alignment, hydrogen atoms broadcast energy in the form of a signal that is received by the antenna and processed by the computer to reconstruct images. The energy of and the time interval between RF pulses and time delays before receiving the signal can be selected and constitute the *pulse sequence.* Signal intensity from a given tissue in the slice determines the shade of gray on a black and white image. In medical imaging, higher signals are assigned lighter (brighter) shades and lower signals darker shades.

Signal intensity depends on three inherent properties of the tissue: the water content in a unit volume of tissue (proton density) and two important magnetic characteristics of the tissue known as relaxation times, T1 (relaxation time 1, shorter) and T2 (relaxation time 2, longer). While a higher water content yields higher (brighter) signals, the water content signal is greatly modulated by the opposing effects of the tissue-dependent relaxation times T1 and T2. T1 or T2 can be selectively emphasized, resulting in T1-weighted or T2-weighted images. T1-weighted images show higher (brighter) signals in white matter than in gray matter and resemble anatomic brain slices. The CSF in T1-weighted images has a low signal and is dark. On the other hand, in T2-weighted images, the signal is low (dark) in white matter, resembling a myelin stain, while the signal in the CSF is high (bright), emphasizing the ventricles, cisterns, and subarachnoid space.

A set of parallel images is obtained in a two-dimensional (2D) or a three-dimensional (3D) mode. In the 2D mode, the RF pulse is delivered to different slices in rapid succession, and the signal is acquired one slice at a time. After the last slice, the process is repeated, typically 192–250 times. A 2D acquisition typically has 20 slices, 5 mm thick. A separate 2D acquisition is required for each plane. In the 3D mode, the RF pulse is delivered to the entire volume, and the slice thickness can be reduced to 1 mm without significant loss of signal-to-noise. Although the 3D acquisition is made in one plane, for example, sagittal, because of the small slice thickness, the data set can be reformatted and viewed in any other plane.

The MRI images in *The Brain Atlas: A Visual Guide to the Human Central Nervous System* were obtained from a normal live human subject in a 1.5 Tesla magnet with a T1-weighted pulse sequence in the 3D mode (MPRAGE by Siemens Corp., Erlangen). Heavy T1 weighting makes the MRIs similar to the brain slices. The data set consisted of 128 sagittal 1-mm sections at a resolution of 1.2 X 1.0 X 1.0 mm, which were reformatted to generate images selected to match the anatomic slices. Differences between the brain slices and the MRIs are due to normal anatomic variations between human brains.

Magnetic Resonance Angiography

Magnetic resonance angiography does not require injection of contrast material into the bloodstream. Unlike MRI, in which the emphasis is on signals from stationary molecules, magnetic resonance angiography emphasizes signals from moving molecules in blood vessels, while signals from molecules in stationary tissues are suppressed. Images of arteries and veins can be separated during data acquisition by using "saturation bands" that nullify signals from molecules within the band. By applying a saturation band over the superior sagittal sinus, venous blood flowing from this sinus is made invisible, while blood flowing through the carotid and vertebral arteries remains visible. The result is a *magnetic resonance arteriogram* (MRA). A saturation band applied over arteries of the neck makes blood within the carotid and vertebral arteries and their intracranial branches invisible, while blood flowing through the dural venous sinuses and their tributaries is visible. The result is a *magnetic resonance venogram* (MRV). As in MRI, the images are from 1-mm thick slices. These can be combined to create projections similar to the views in conventional angiography.

References

Brodal A: Neurological Anatomy in Relation to Clinical Medicine, ed 2. New York, Oxford University Press, 1981.

Brodmann K: Vergleichende Lokalisationslehre der Grosshirnrinde in ihren Prinzipien dargestellt auf Grund des Zellenbaues. Leipzig, JA Barth, 1909.

Duvernoy HM: The Human Brain: Surface, Three-Dimensional Sectional Anatomy and MRI. New York, Springer-Verlag, 1991.

Duvernoy HM: The Human Hippocampus: An Atlas of Applied Anatomy. Munich, JF Bergmann Verlag, 1988.

Duvernoy HM: Human Brain Stem Vessels. Berlin, Springer-Verlag, 1978.

Gabe M: Histological Techniques. Paris, Masson, 1976.

Haymaker W, Anderson E, Nauta WJH: The Hypothalamus. Springfield, Ill., Thomas, 1969.

Lasjaunias P, Berenstein A: Surgical Neuroangiography: 3. Functional Vascular Anatomy of Brain, Spinal Cord and Spine. Berlin, Springer-Verlag, 1990.

Loewy AD, Spyer KM: Central Regulation of Autonomic Functions. New York, Oxford University Press, 1990.

Mulligan JH: A method of staining the brain for macroscopic study. J Anat 65:468-472, 1931.

Nieuwenhuys R: Chemoarchitecture of the Brain. New York, Springer-Verlag, 1985.

Nieuwenhuys R, Voogd J, van Huijzen C: The Human Central Nervous System: A Synopsis and Atlas. New York, Springer-Verlag, 1988.

Olszewski J, Baxter D: Cytoarchitecture of the Human Brain Stem. Philadelphia, Lippincott, 1954.

Paxinos G: The Human Nervous System. San Diego, Academic Press, 1990.

Posner MI, Raichle ME: Images of Mind. New York, Scientific American, 1994.

Rasmussen AT: The Principal Nervous Pathways: Neurological Charts and Schemas, with Explanatory Notes. New York, Macmillan, 1932.

Riley HA: An Atlas of the Basal Ganglia, Brain Stem and Spinal Cord: Based on Myelin-Stained Material. Baltimore, Williams and Wilkins, 1943.

Roberts MP, Hanaway J, Morest DK: Atlas of the Human Brain in Section, ed 2. Philadelphia, Lea and Febiger, 1987.

Salamon G: Atlas of the Arteries of the Human Brain. Paris, Sandoz, 1971.

Schaltenbrand G, Bailey P: Introduction to Stereotaxis with an Atlas of the Human Brain. 3 Volumes. Stuttgart, Georg Thieme Verlag, 1959.

Szikla G, Bouvier G, Hori T, Petrov V: Angiography of the Human Brain Cortex: Atlas of Vascular Patterns and Stereotactic Cortical Localization. Berlin, Springer-Verlag, 1977.

Talairach J, Tournoux P: Co-planar Stereotaxic Atlas of the Human Brain: 3-dimensional Proportional System: An Approach to Cerebral Imaging. New York, Thieme Medical Publishers, 1988.

Van Buren JM, Borke RC: Variations and Connections of the Human Thalamus. 2 Vols. New York, Springer-Verlag, 1972.

The Brain and Its Blood Vessels

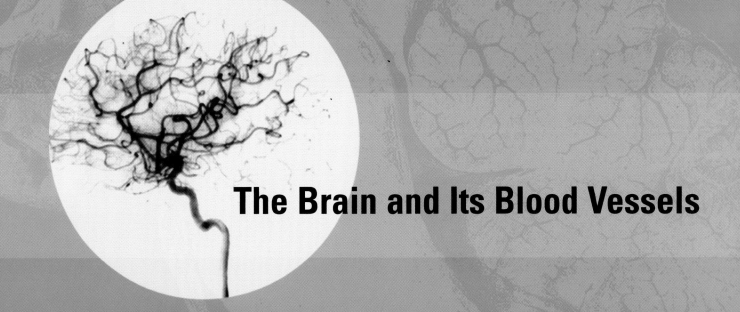

Part II

The Brain and Its Blood Vessels

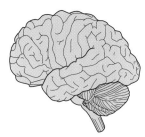

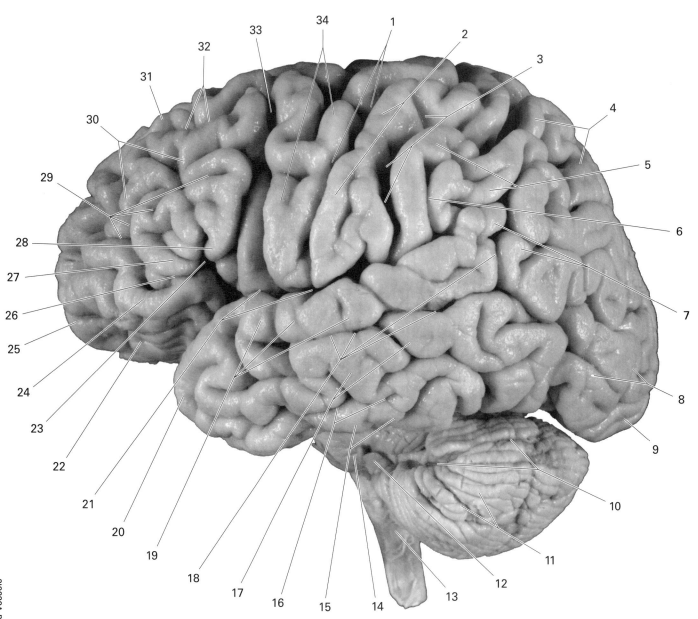

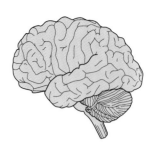

1 Central sulcus (fissure of *Rolando*)
2 Postcentral gyrus
3 Postcentral sulcus
4 Superior parietal lobule
5 Supramarginal gyrus
6 Lateral sulcus *(Sylvian* fissure), posterior ascending limb (ramus)
7 Angular gyrus
8 Lateral occipital gyri
9 Occipital pole
10 Cerebellum, horizontal fissure
11 Cerebellum, hemisphere
12 Cerebellum, flocculus
13 Medulla oblongata
14 Pons
15 Inferior temporal gyrus
16 Inferior temporal sulcus
17 Middle temporal gyrus
18 Superior temporal sulcus
19 Superior temporal gyrus
20 Temporal pole
21 Lateral sulcus (*Sylvian* fissure), posterior horizontal limb (ramus)
22 Orbital gyri
23 Lateral sulcus (*Sylvian* fissure), anterior ascending limb (ramus)
24 Inferior frontal gyrus, orbital part
25 Frontal pole
26 Lateral sulcus (*Sylvian* fissure), anterior horizontal limb (ramus)
27 Inferior frontal gyrus, triangular part
28 Inferior frontal gyrus, opercular part
29 Inferior frontal sulcus
30 Middle frontal gyrus
31 Superior frontal gyrus
32 Superior frontal sulcus
33 Precentral sulcus
34 Precentral gyrus

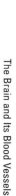

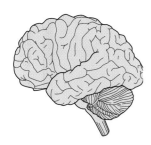

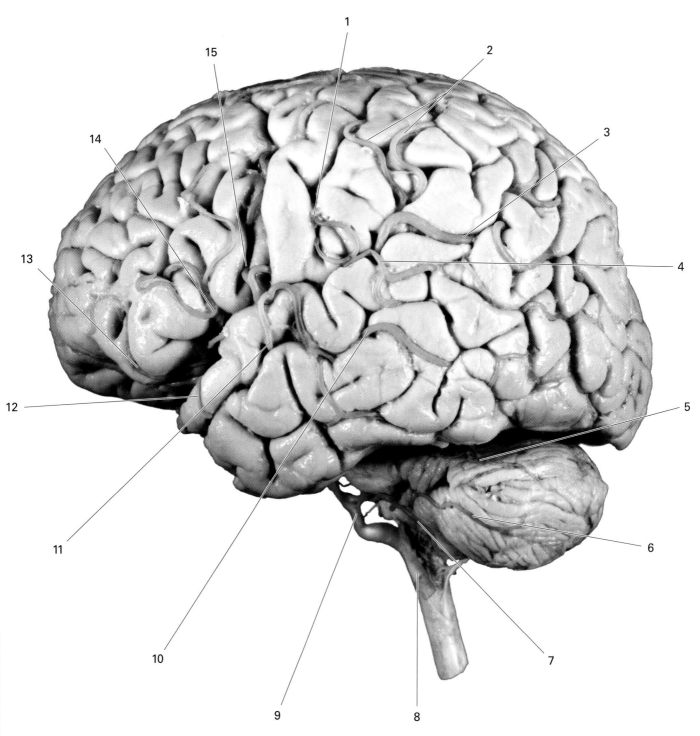

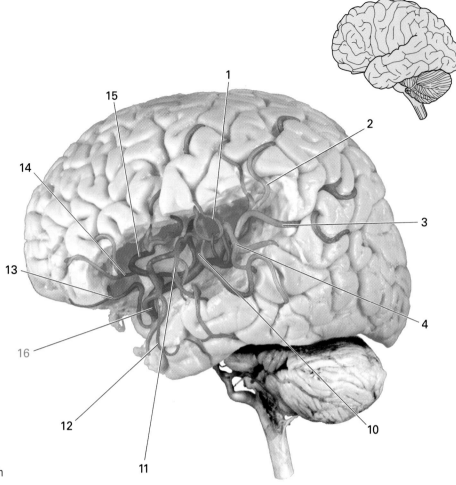

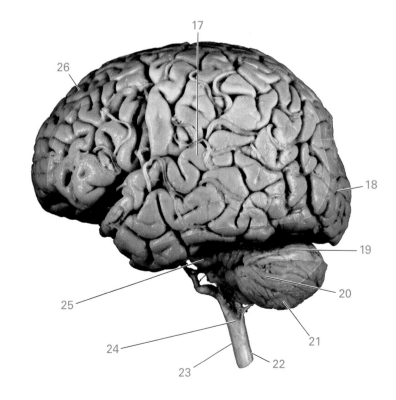

1	Middle cerebral artery, central sulcus branch
2	Middle cerebral artery, parietal branch
3	Middle cerebral artery, angular branch
4	Middle cerebral artery, posterior temporal branch
5	Superior cerebellar artery
6	Anterior inferior cerebellar artery
7	Posterior inferior cerebellar artery
8	Vertebral artery
9	Basilar artery
10	Middle cerebral artery, middle temporal branch
11	Middle cerebral artery, anterior temporal branch
12	Middle cerebral artery, temporopolar branch
13	Middle cerebral artery, orbital branch
14	Middle cerebral artery, orbitofrontal branch
15	Middle cerebral artery, operculofrontal branch
16	Middle cerebral artery, stem
17	Middle cerebral artery territory
18	Posterior cerebral artery territory
19	Superior cerebellar artery territory
20	Anterior inferior cerebellar artery territory
21	Posterior inferior cerebellar artery territory
22	Posterior spinal artery territory
23	Anterior spinal artery territory
24	Vertebral artery territory
25	Basilar artery, lateral branches territory
26	Anterior cerebral artery territory

The Brain and Its Blood Vessels

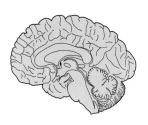

Cerebral Hemisphere and Brain Stem (1X)–Mesial Aspect

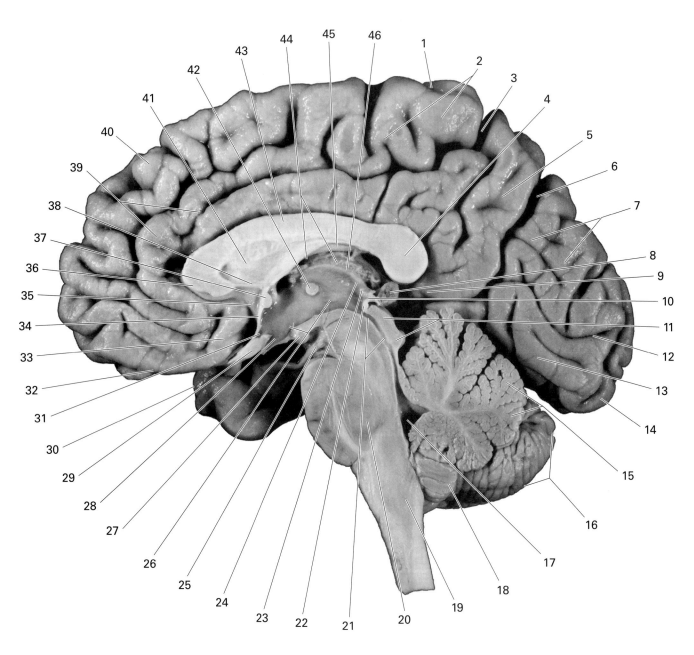

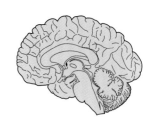

1	Central sulcus (fissure of *Rolando*)
2	Paracentral lobule
3	Cingulate sulcus, marginal branch
4	Corpus callosum, splenium
5	Parietal lobe, precuneus
6	Parieto-occipital sulcus
7	Occipital lobe, cuneus
8	Pineal gland
9	Cingulate gyrus, isthmus
10	Third ventricle (III), pineal recess
11	Superior and inferior colliculi (quadrigeminal plate, tectum)
12	Calcarine fissure
13	Medial occipitotemporal (lingual) gyrus
14	Occipital pole
15	Cerebellum, vermis
16	Cerebellum, hemisphere
17	Fourth ventricle (IV)
18	Cerebellum, tonsil (ventral paraflocculus)
19	Medulla oblongata
20	Pons
21	Cerebral aqueduct (aqueduct of *Sylvius*)
22	Posterior commissure
23	Habenular commissure
24	Habenula
25	Oculomotor nerve (CN III)
26	Third ventricle (III)
27	Mamillary body
28	Third ventricle (III), infundibular recess
29	Optic chiasm
30	Temporal pole
31	Third ventricle (III), optic recess
32	Gyrus rectus (straight gyrus)
33	Subcallosal area
34	Lamina terminalis
35	Preterminal gyrus
36	Corpus callosum, genu
37	Anterior commissure
38	Corpus callosum, rostrum
39	Cingulate sulcus and gyrus
40	Superior frontal gyrus
41	Septum pellucidum
42	Interthalamic adhesion (massa intermedia)
43	Corpus callosum, body
44	Choroid plexus of lateral ventricle and interventricular foramen (of *Monro*)
45	Fornix, body
46	Stria medullaris of thalamus

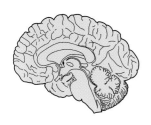

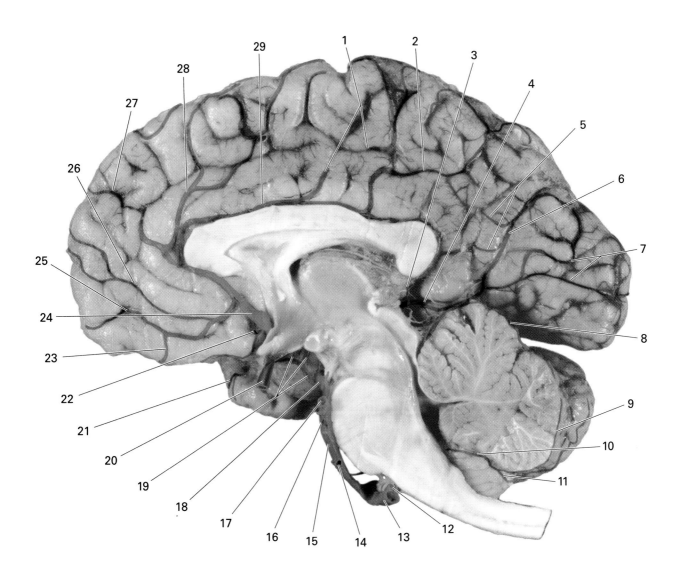

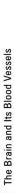

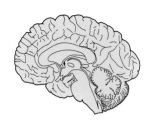

1	Anterior cerebral artery, callosomarginal branch
2	Anterior cerebral artery, pericallosal artery
3	Medial posterior choroidal artery
4	Posterior cerebral artery
5	Posterior cerebral artery, parieto-occipital branch, precuneal branches
6	Posterior cerebral artery, parieto-occipital branch
7	Posterior cerebral artery, calcarine branch
8	Superior cerebellar artery
9	Posterior inferior cerebellar artery, vermian branch
10	Posterior inferior cerebellar artery
11	Posterior inferior cerebellar artery, tonsillohemispheric branch
12	Posterior inferior cerebellar artery, origin
13	Vertebral artery
14	Anterior inferior cerebellar artery, origin
15	Basilar artery
16	Superior cerebellar artery, origin
17	Posterior cerebral artery, origin
18	Posterior cerebral artery
19	Posterior communicating artery and perforating branches
20	Internal carotid artery
21	Middle cerebral artery, temporopolar branch
22	Anterior communicating artery
23	Anterior cerebral artery, orbital branch
24	Anterior cerebral artery
25	Anterior cerebral artery, frontopolar branch
26	Anterior cerebral artery, anterior internal frontal branch
27	Anterior cerebral artery, middle internal frontal branch
28	Anterior cerebral artery, posterior internal frontal branch
29	Anterior cerebral artery, pericallosal arteries
30	Choroidal arteries territory
31	Posterior cerebral artery territory
32	Posterior cerebral artery, collicular and posterior medial choroidal branches territory
33	Superior cerebellar artery territory
34	Posterior inferior cerebellar artery territory
35	Posterior spinal artery territory
36	Anterior spinal artery territory
37	Basilar artery, medial branches territory
38	Posterior cerebral artery, perforating branches territory
39	Posterior cerebral artery territory

40	Internal carotid artery territory
41	Middle cerebral artery territory
42	Anterior cerebral artery territory
43	Posterior communicating artery territory
44	Anterior cerebral artery territory

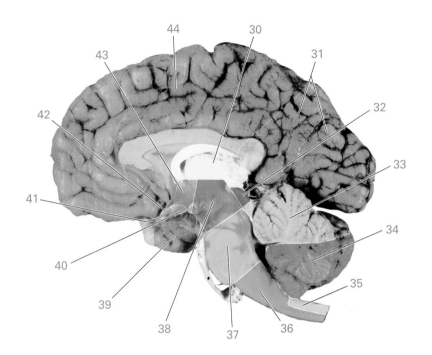

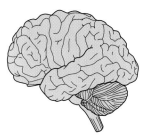

Cerebral Hemisphere and Brain Stem Arteries by Conventional Radiography (0.7X); by MRA (1X)–Lateral Projection

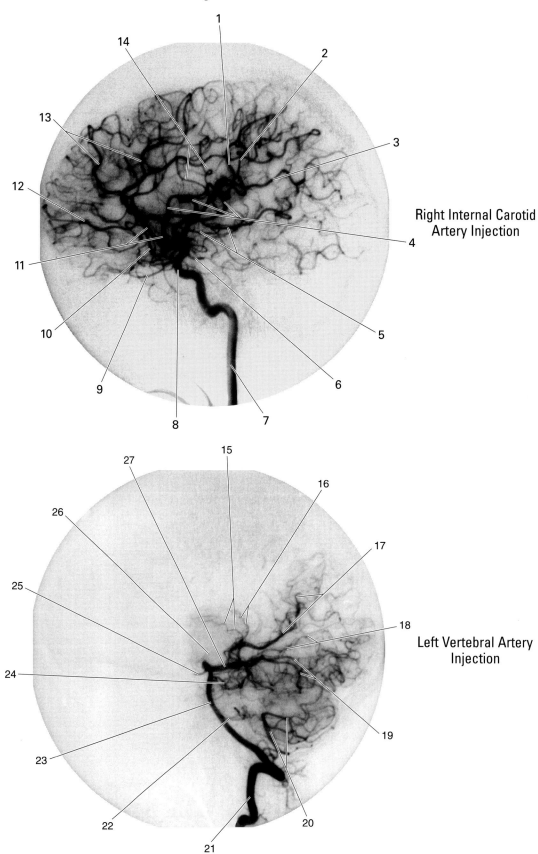

Right Internal Carotid Artery Injection

Left Vertebral Artery Injection

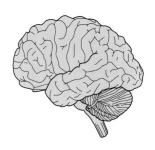

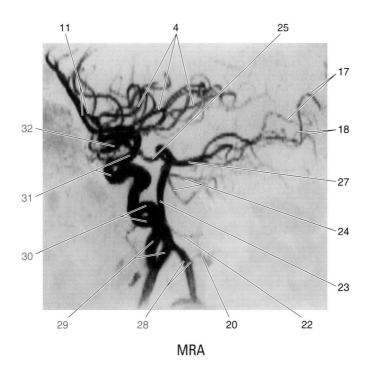

MRA

1	Middle cerebral artery, central sulcus branch
2	Middle cerebral artery, parietal branches
3	Middle cerebral artery, angular branch
4	Middle cerebral artery, branches on insula
5	Middle cerebral artery, temporal branches
6	Posterior communicating artery
7	Internal carotid artery, extracranial part
8	Internal carotid artery, carotid siphon (intracavernous part)
9	Ophthalmic artery
10	Middle cerebral artery, orbitofrontal branch
11	Anterior cerebral arteries, pericallosal arteries
12	Anterior cerebral artery, frontopolar branch
13	Anterior cerebral artery, internal frontal branches
14	Middle cerebral artery, operculofrontal branches
15	Medial posterior choroidal arteries
16	Lateral posterior choroidal arteries
17	Posterior cerebral artery, parieto-occipital branch
18	Posterior cerebral artery, calcarine branch
19	Posterior cerebral artery, posterior temporal branches
20	Posterior inferior cerebellar arteries
21	Vertebral artery
22	Anterior inferior cerebellar arteries
23	Basilar artery
24	Superior cerebellar arteries
25	Posterior communicating artery
26	Posterior cerebral arteries, perforating branches
27	Posterior cerebral arteries
28	Vertebral arteries (superimposed)
29	Internal carotid arteries, extracranial parts (superimposed)
30	Internal carotid arteries, intrapetrous parts (superimposed)
31	Internal carotid arteries, carotid siphons (intracavernous parts) (superimposed)
32	Middle cerebral artery, stem

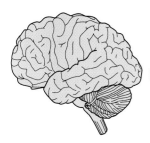

Dural Venous Sinuses and Folds (Diagrammatic, 0.7X); by Conventional Radiography (0.7X); by MRV (0.7X)–Lateral Projection

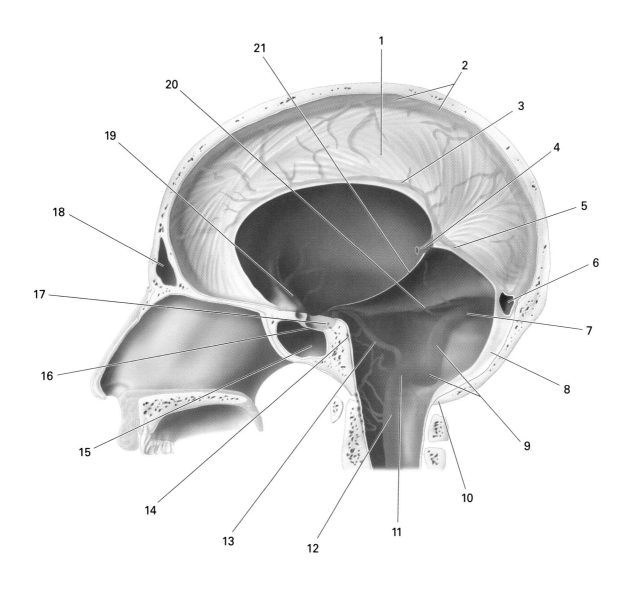

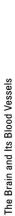

1	Falx cerebri
2	Superior sagittal sinus
3	Inferior sagittal sinus
4	Great cerebral vein (vein of *Galen*)
5	Straight sinus
6	Confluence of dural venous sinuses (torcular of *Herophilus*)
7	Transverse sinus
8	Falx cerebelli
9	Sigmoid sinus
10	Foramen magnum, posterior rim
11	Jugular bulb
12	Internal jugular vein
13	Inferior petrosal sinus
14	Clival venous plexus
15	Sphenoidal air sinus
16	Sella turcica
17	Cavernous sinus
18	Frontal air sinus
19	Sphenoparietal sinus
20	Superior petrosal sinus
21	Tentorium cerebelli
22	Superior cerebral veins
23	Lateral occipital veins
24	Inferior anastomotic vein (vein of *Labbé*)
25	Basal vein (basal vein of *Rosenthal*)
26	Internal cerebral vein
27	Septal vein
28	Superior cerebral veins
29	Thalamostriate vein
30	Anterior caudate vein

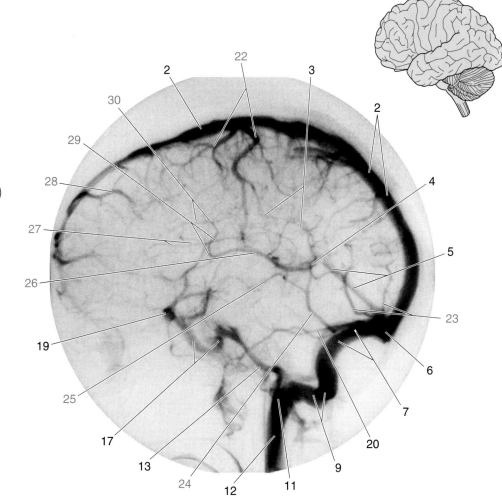

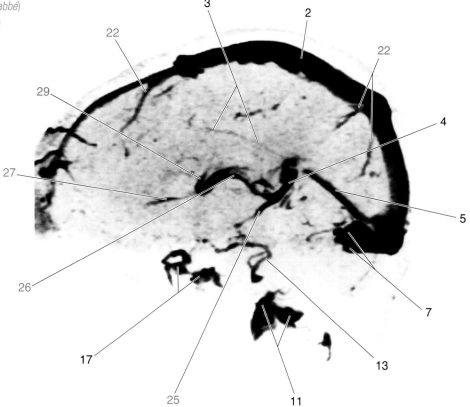

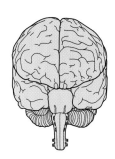

Cerebral Hemispheres, Brain Stem, and Arteries (1X); by MRA (1X)–Anterior Aspect

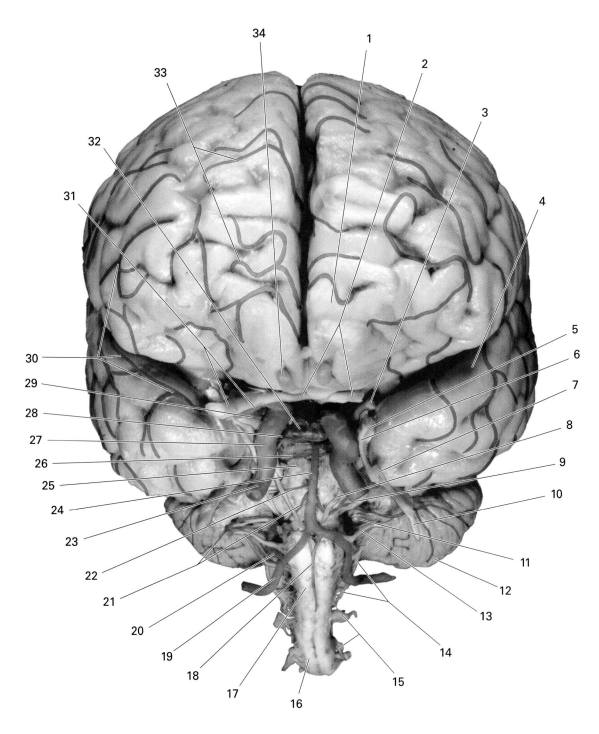

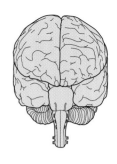

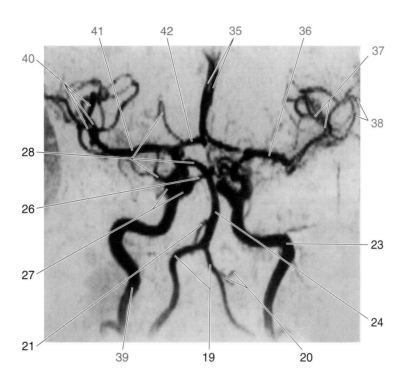

1	Frontal pole
2	Optic chiasm and optic nerve (CN II)
3	Oculomotor nerve (CN III)
4	Temporal lobe
5	Trigeminal nerve (CN V), ophthalmic division (V1)
6	Abducent nerve (CN VI)
7	Trigeminal nerve (CN V), maxillary division (V2)
8	Abducent nerve (CN VI)
9	Facial and vestibulocochlear nerves (CN VII and CN VIII)
10	Trigeminal nerve (CN V), mandibular division (V3)
11	Glossopharyngeal and vagus nerves (CN IX and CN X)
12	Cerebellum, hemisphere
13	Hypoglossal nerve (CN XII)
14	Accessory nerve (CN XI)
15	Spinal nerves (C1 and C2)
16	Spinal cord
17	Medulla oblongata
18	Anterior spinal artery
19	Vertebral artery
20	Posterior inferior cerebellar artery
21	Anterior inferior cerebellar artery
22	Basilar artery, lateral branch

23	Internal carotid artery, intrapetrous part
24	Basilar artery
25	Pons
26	Superior cerebellar artery
27	Internal carotid artery, carotid siphon (intracavernous part)
28	Posterior cerebral artery
29	Trochlear nerve (CN IV)
30	Middle cerebral artery, branches
31	Optic nerve (CN II) and ophthalmic artery
32	Pituitary gland
33	Anterior cerebral artery, branches
34	Olfactory bulb
35	Anterior cerebral arteries, pericallosal arteries
36	Middle cerebral artery, stem
37	Middle cerebral artery, branches on insula
38	Middle cerebral artery, branches on hemispheric convexity
39	Internal carotid artery, extracranial part
40	Middle cerebral artery, branches on insula
41	Middle cerebral artery, stem
42	Anterior cerebral artery

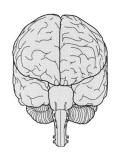

Cerebral Hemisphere and Brain Stem Arteries and Veins by Conventional Radiography (0.7X)– Anteroposterior Projection

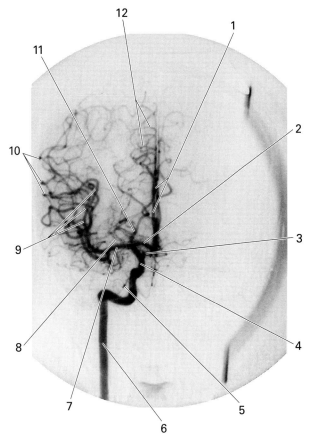

Right Internal Carotid Artery Injection

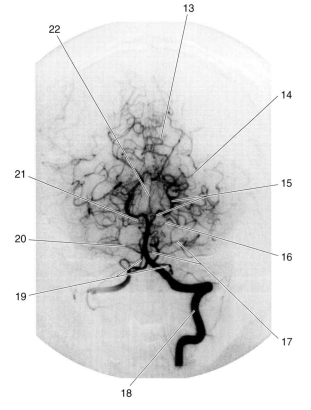

Left Vertebral Artery Injection

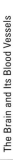

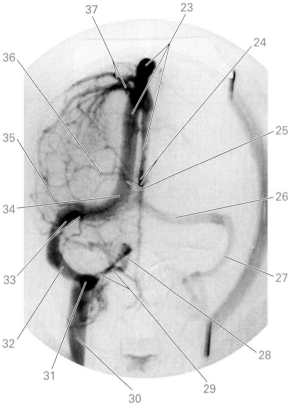

1	Anterior cerebral arteries, pericallosal arteries
2	Anterior cerebral artery
3	Posterior communicating artery
4	Internal carotid artery, carotid siphon (intracavernous part)
5	Ophthalmic artery
6	Internal carotid artery, extracranial part
7	Middle cerebral artery, stem
8	Middle cerebral artery, lateral lenticulostriate branches
9	Middle cerebral artery, branches on insula
10	Middle cerebral artery, branches on hemispheric convexity
11	Posterior cerebral artery
12	Anterior cerebral artery, pericallosal artery branches
13	Posterior cerebral artery, calcarine branch
14	Posterior cerebral artery, posterior temporal branch
15	Posterior cerebral artery
16	Superior cerebellar artery
17	Anterior inferior cerebellar artery
18	Vertebral artery
19	Posterior inferior cerebellar arteries
20	Anterior inferior cerebellar artery
21	Posterior communicating artery
22	Posterior inferior cerebellar arteries, vermian branches
23	Superior sagittal sinus
24	Internal cerebral vein and great cerebral vein (vein of *Galen*)
25	Thalamostriate vein
26	Transverse sinus
27	Sigmoid sinus
28	Cavernous sinus
29	Inferior petrosal sinus
30	Internal jugular vein
31	Jugular bulb
32	Sigmoid sinus
33	Transverse sinus
34	Confluence of dural venous sinuses (torcular of *Herophilus*)
35	Inferior anastomotic vein (vein of *Labbé*)
36	Lateral occipital veins
37	Superior cerebral veins

Right Internal Carotid Artery Injection

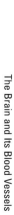

The Brain and Its Blood Vessels

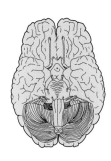

Cerebral Hemispheres and Brain Stem (1X);
Arteries (0.7X)–Inferior Aspect

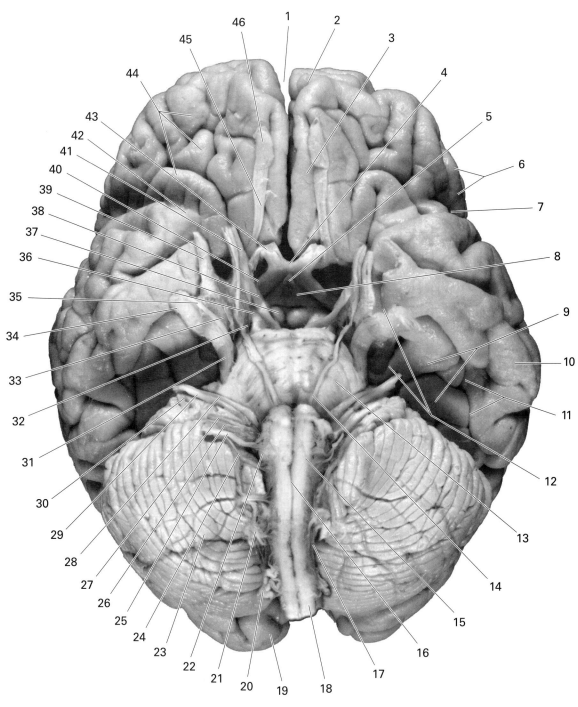

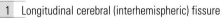

1 Longitudinal cerebral (interhemispheric) fissure
2 Frontal pole
3 Gyrus rectus (straight gyrus)
4 Optic chiasm
5 Infundibulum (pituitary stalk)
6 Inferior frontal gyrus
7 Lateral sulcus (*Sylvian* fissure), stem
8 Tuber cinereum
9 Lateral occipitotemporal gyrus (fusiform gyrus)
10 Inferior temporal gyrus
11 Occipitotemporal sulcus
12 Collateral sulcus
13 Pons
14 Abducent nerve (CN VI)
15 Pyramid (corticospinal tract)
16 Medulla oblongata, anterior median fissure
17 Accessory nerve (CN XI), spinal root
18 Spinal cord
19 Occipital pole
20 Spinal nerve (C3)
21 Spinal nerve (C2)
22 Inferior olive
23 Cerebellum, hemisphere
24 Accessory nerve (CN XI)
25 Hypoglossal nerve (CN XII)
26 Vagus nerve (CN X)
27 Glossopharyngeal nerve (CN IX)
28 Facial nerve (CN VII)
29 Vestibulocochlear nerve (CN VIII)
30 Cerebellum, flocculus
31 Trigeminal nerve (CN V), sensory root
32 Trochlear nerve (CN IV)
33 Trigeminal (CN V) ganglion
34 Trigeminal nerve (CN V), mandibular division (V3)
35 Trigeminal nerve (CN V), motor root
36 Cerebral peduncle
37 Mamillary body
38 Oculomotor nerve (CN III)
39 Trigeminal nerve (CN V), maxillary division (V2)
40 Optic tract
41 Trigeminal nerve (CN V), ophthalmic division (V1)
42 Temporal pole
43 Optic nerve (CN II)
44 Orbital gyri
45 Olfactory tract
46 Olfactory bulb

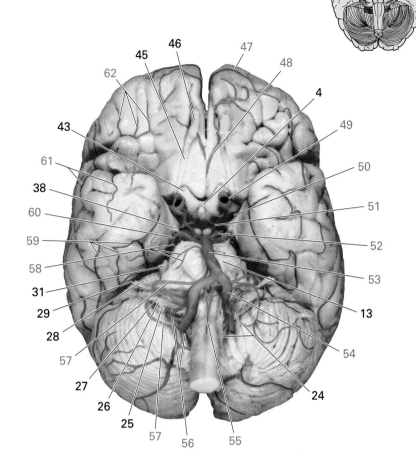

47 Anterior cerebral artery, frontopolar branch
48 Anterior cerebral artery, orbital branch
49 Internal carotid artery
50 Anterior choroidal artery
51 Posterior communicating artery
52 Posterior cerebral artery
53 Basilar artery
54 Vertebral artery
55 Anterior spinal artery
56 Posterior inferior cerebellar artery
57 Anterior inferior cerebellar artery
58 Basilar artery, lateral branches
59 Posterior cerebral artery, posterior temporal branches
60 Superior cerebellar artery
61 Middle cerebral artery, temporopolar branches
62 Middle cerebral artery, orbital branches

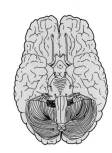

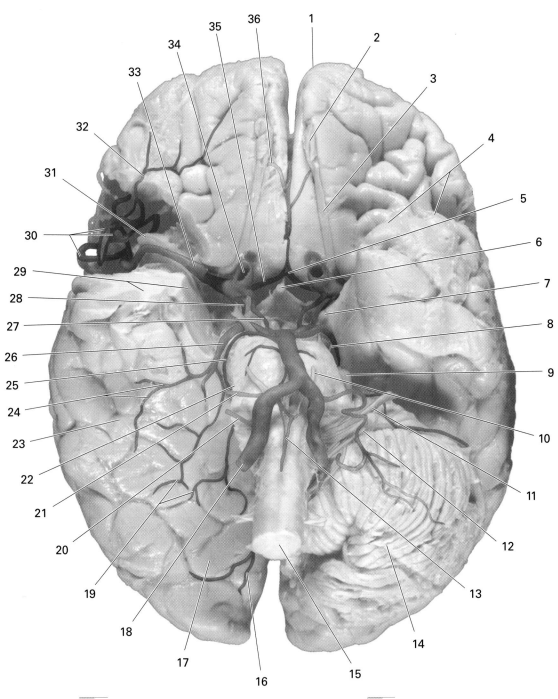

1	Frontal pole	6	Infundibulum (pituitary stalk)
2	Olfactory bulb	7	Oculomotor nerve (CN III)
3	Olfactory tract	8	Trochlear nerve (CN IV)
4	Temporal pole	9	Trigeminal nerve (CN V), sensory root
5	Anterior communicating artery	10	Abducent nerve (CN VI)

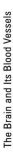

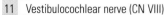

11	Vestibulocochlear nerve (CN VIII)
12	Accessory nerve (CN XI)
13	Anterior spinal artery
14	Cerebellum, hemisphere
15	Spinal cord, cut surface
16	Posterior cerebral artery, calcarine branch
17	Occipital lobe
18	Vertebral artery
19	Posterior cerebral artery, posterior temporal branches
20	Posterior inferior cerebellar artery
21	Anterior inferior cerebellar artery
22	Middle cerebellar peduncle (brachium pontis), cut surface
23	Temporal lobe
24	Posterior cerebral artery, posterior temporal branches
25	Superior cerebellar artery
26	Posterior cerebral artery
27	Posterior communicating artery
28	Anterior choroidal artery
29	Temporal lobe, cut surfaces
30	Middle cerebral artery, branches on insula
31	Insula
32	Middle cerebral artery, orbital branch
33	Middle cerebral artery, stem
34	Internal carotid artery
35	Anterior cerebral artery
36	Anterior cerebral artery, orbital branch
37	Anterior cerebral artery territory
38	Ophthalmic artery territory
39	Middle cerebral artery territory
40	Internal carotid artery territory
41	Anterior choroidal artery territory
42	Posterior communicating artery territory
43	Posterior cerebral artery territory
44	Superior cerebellar artery territory
45	Basilar artery, lateral branches territory
46	Basilar artery, medial branches territory
47	Anterior inferior cerebellar artery territory
48	Posterior inferior cerebellar artery territory
49	Vertebral artery territory
50	Anterior spinal artery territory
51	Anterior cerebral arteries, pericallosal arteries
52	Middle cerebral artery, branches on hemispheric convexity
53	Basilar artery
54	Posterior cerebral artery, calcarine branch
55	Internal carotid artery, intrapetrous part
56	Internal carotid artery, carotid siphon (intracavernous part)
57	Ophthalmic artery

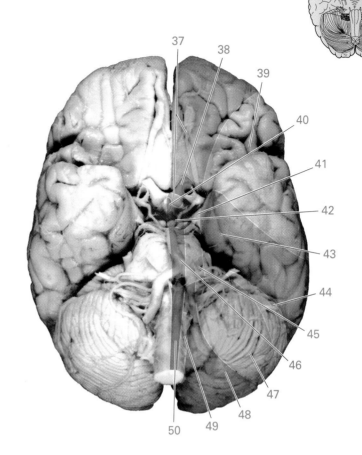

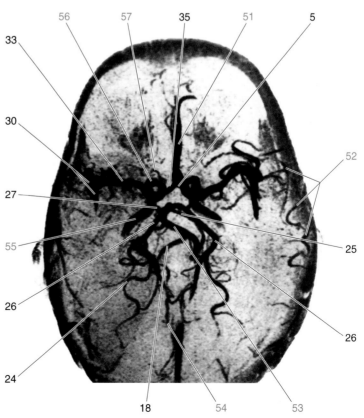

The Brain and Its Blood Vessels

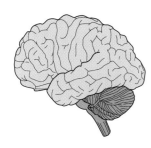

Brain Stem, Diencephalon, Basal Ganglia, and Cerebellum (1X); Arteries (0.6X); Arterial Territories (0.6X)–Anterolateral Aspect

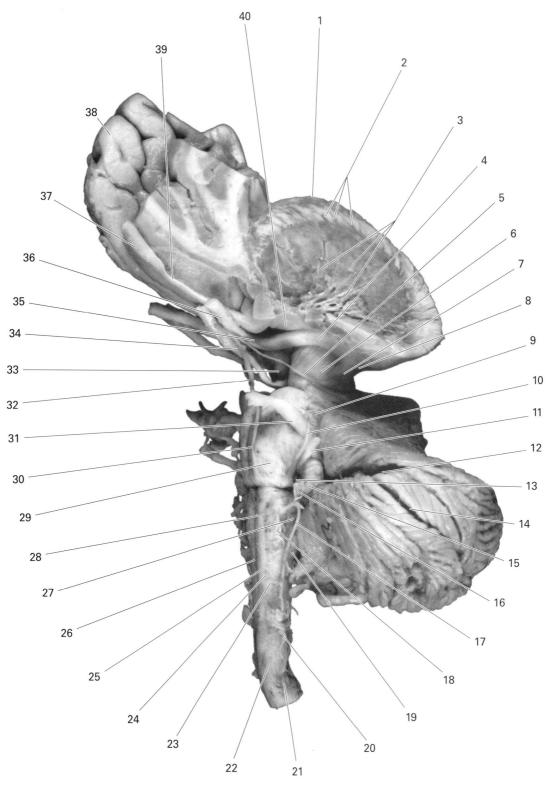

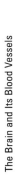

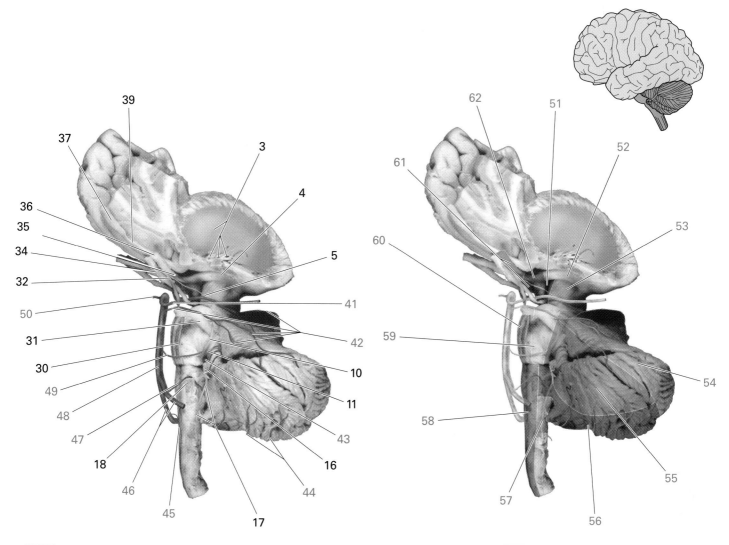

1	Caudate nucleus, body
2	Caudatolenticular gray bridges
3	Putamen and middle cerebral artery, lateral lenticulostriate branches
4	Optic tract
5	Trochlear nerve (CN IV)
6	Cerebral peduncle
7	Thalamus, medial geniculate nucleus (MG) (medial geniculate body)
8	Thalamus, dorsal lateral geniculate nucleus (dLGN) (lateral geniculate body)
9	Middle cerebellar peduncle (brachium pontis)
10	Facial nerve (CN VII)
11	Vestibulocochlear nerve (CN VIII)
12	Cerebellum, primary fissure
13	Choroid plexus and lateral aperture (foramen of *Luschka*) of fourth ventricle (IV)
14	Cerebellum, horizontal fissure
15	Cerebellum, flocculus
16	Glossopharyngeal and vagus nerves (CN IX and CN X)
17	Accessory nerve (CN XI)
18	Hypoglossal nerve (CN XII)
19	Inferior olive
20	Spinal nerve (C2)

21	Spinal nerve (C3)
22	Spinal cord
23	Lateral funiculus
24	Anterolateral (ventrolateral) sulcus
25	Anterior funiculus
26	Anterior (ventral) median fissure (sulcus)
27	Inferior cerebellar peduncle (restiform body)
28	Pyramid (corticospinal tract)
29	Pons
30	Abducent nerve (CN VI)
31	Trigeminal nerve (CN V)
32	Abducent nerve (CN VI)
33	Mamillary body
34	Oculomotor nerve (CN III)
35	Optic chiasm
36	Optic nerve (CN II)
37	Olfactory bulb
38	Frontal pole
39	Olfactory tract
40	Anterior perforated substance
41	Posterior cerebral artery (IV)
42	Superior cerebellar artery and branches
43	Choroid plexus and lateral aperature (foramen of *Luschka*) of fourth ventricle (IV)

44	Posterior inferior cerebellar artery, hemispheric branches
45	Anterior spinal artery
46	Vertebral arteries
47	Posterior inferior cerebellar artery
48	Basilar artery
49	Anterior inferior cerebellar artery
50	Posterior communicating artery
51	Posterior cerebral artery, perforating branches territory
52	Choroidal arteries territory
53	Posterior cerebral artery, collicular and posterior medial choroidal branches territory
54	Superior cerebellar artery territory
55	Anterior inferior cerebellar artery territory
56	Posterior inferior cerebellar artery territory
57	Vertebral artery territory
58	Anterior spinal artery territory
59	Basilar artery, lateral branches territory
60	Basilar artery, medial branches territory
61	Internal carotid artery territory
62	Anterior cerebral artery territory

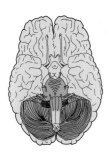

Cerebellum (1X)–Superior Surface

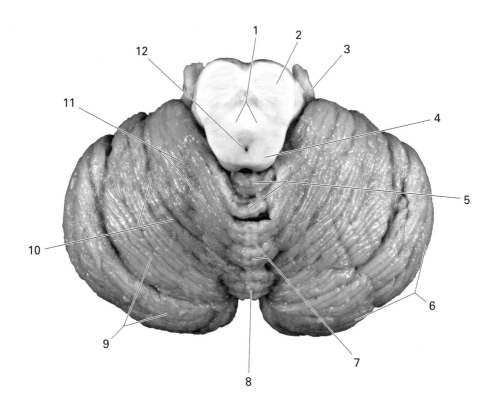

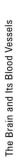
1	Superior cerebellar peduncle, decussation
2	Pons, basilar part (basis pontis)
3	Trigeminal nerve (CN V)
4	Inferior colliculus
5	Cerebellum, vermis, central lobule
6	Cerebellum, hemisphere

7	Cerebellum, vermis, culmen
8	Cerebellum, vermis, declive
9	Cerebellum, posterior lobe
10	Cerebellum, primary fissure
11	Cerebellum, anterior lobe
12	Cerebral aqueduct (aqueduct of *Sylvius*)

Cerebellum (1X)–Inferior Surface

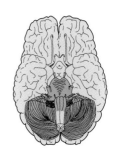

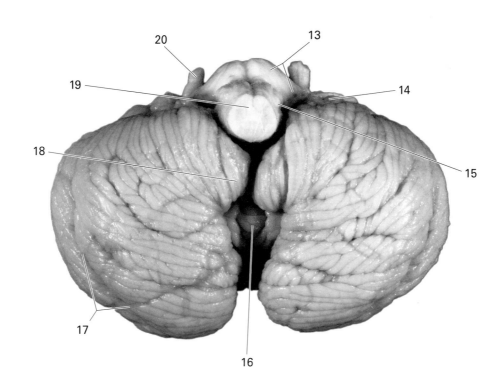

13	Pons and middle cerebellar peduncle (brachium pontis)
14	Cerebellum, flocculus
15	Inferior olive
16	Cerebellum, vermis, nodule
17	Cerebellum, horizontal fissure
18	Cerebellum, tonsil
19	Pyramidal decussation (corticospinal tracts)
20	Trigeminal nerve (CN V)

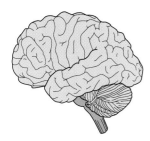

Brain Stem, Thalamus, and Striatum (1X)–Anterior, Posterior, and Lateral Aspects

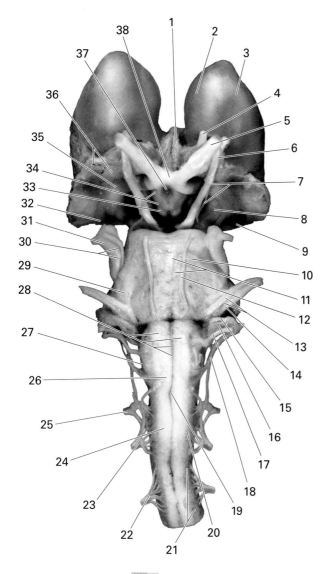

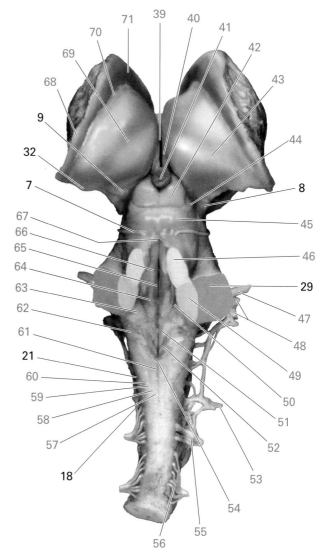

1	Fornix, column	13	Facial nerve (CN VII)
2	Caudate nucleus, head	14	Vestibulocochlear nerve (CN VIII)
3	Putamen	15	Glossopharyngeal nerve (CN IX)
4	Olfactory tract	16	Vagus nerve (CN X)
5	Optic nerve (CN II)	17	Hypoglossal nerve (CN XII)
6	Oculomotor nerve (CN III)	18	Accessory nerve (CN XI)
7	Trochlear nerve (CN IV)	19	Anterior (ventral) median fissure (sulcus)
8	Cerebral peduncle	20	Spinal cord, anterior lateral sulcus
9	Thalamus, medial geniculate nucleus (MG) (medial geniculate body)	21	Lateral funiculus
		22	Spinal nerve (C3)
10	Pons	23	Spinal nerve (C2)
11	Basilar sulcus of pons	24	Anterior funiculus
12	Abducent nerve (CN VI)	25	Spinal nerve (C1)

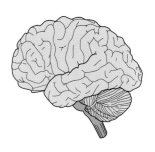

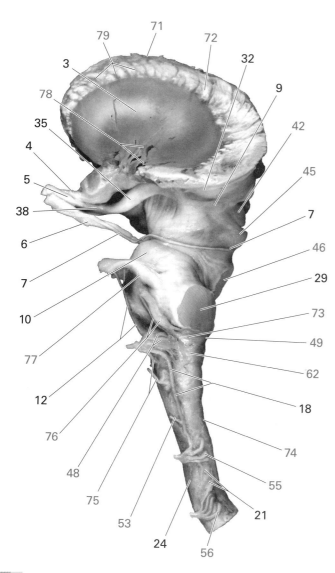

37	Infundibulum (pituitary stalk)
38	Optic chiasm
39	Third ventricle (III)
40	Stria medullaris of thalamus
41	Pineal gland
42	Superior colliculus
43	Thalamus, pulvinar (Pul)
44	Inferior colliculus, brachium
45	Inferior colliculus
46	Superior cerebellar peduncle (brachium conjunctivum)
47	Facial and vestibulocochlear nerves (CN VII and CN VIII)
48	Glossopharyngeal and vagus nerves (CN IX and CN X)
49	Inferior cerebellar peduncle (restiform body)
50	Sulcus limitans
51	Hypoglossal (CN XII) trigone
52	Vagal (CN X) trigone
53	Spinal nerve (C1), anterior (ventral) root (ramus)
54	Obex
55	Spinal nerve (C2), posterior (dorsal) root (ramus)
56	Spinal nerve (C3), posterior (dorsal) root (ramus)
57	Gracile fasciculus
58	Posterior intermediate sulcus
59	Cuneate fasciculus
60	Posterior lateral sulcus
61	Posterior median sulcus
62	Trigeminal tubercle
63	Vestibular area
64	Facial colliculus
65	Median sulcus of fourth ventricle (IV)
66	Medial eminence
67	Superior medullary velum
68	Corona radiata
69	Thalamus
70	Stria terminalis
71	Caudate nucleus, body
72	Internal capsule, posterior limb
73	Cochlear nuclei (CN VIII)
74	Posterior funiculus
75	Hypoglossal nerve (CN XII)
76	Facial and vestibulocochlear nerves (CN VII and CN VIII)
77	Trigeminal nerve (CN V)
78	Middle cerebral artery, lateral lenticulostriate branches
79	Caudatolenticular gray bridges

26	Medulla oblongata
27	Inferior olive
28	Pyramids and pyramidal decussation (corticospinal tract)
29	Middle cerebellar peduncle (brachium pontis)
30	Trigeminal nerve (CN V), motor root
31	Trigeminal nerve (CN V), sensory root
32	Thalamus, dorsal lateral geniculate nucleus (dLGN) (lateral geniculate body)
33	Mamillary body
34	Tuber cinereum
35	Optic tract
36	Anterior perforated substance

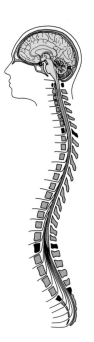

Arteries to Spinal Cord (Diagrammatic)

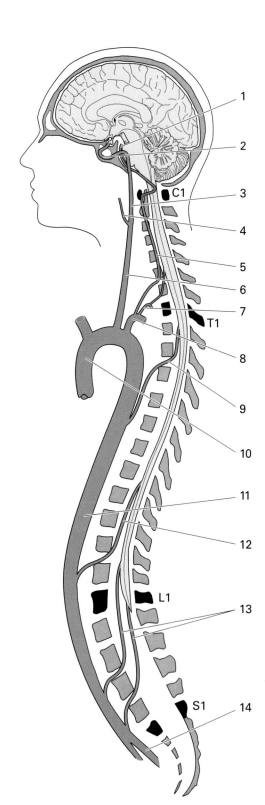

1   Basilar artery
2   Internal carotid artery, carotid siphon
    (intracavernous part)
3   Internal carotid artery
4   External carotid artery
5   Vertebral artery
6   Common carotid artery
7   Thyrocervical trunk
8   Subclavian artery
9   Radicular artery
10 Ascending aorta
11 Descending aorta
12 Radicular artery (of *Adamkiewicz*)
13 Radicular arteries
14 Common iliac artery

Segmental Arterial Supply of Spinal Cord (Diagrammatic)

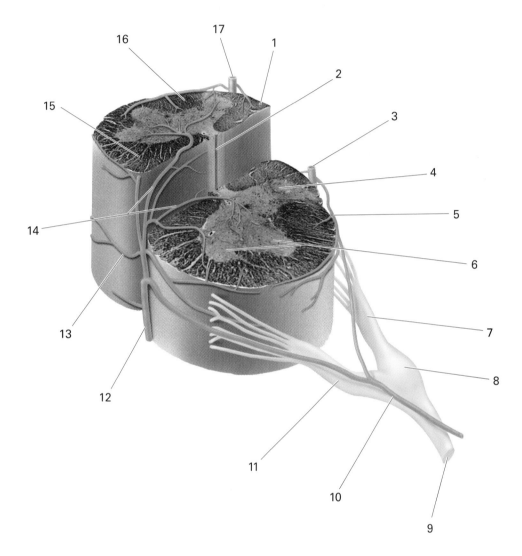

1	Posterior funiculus	10	Radicular artery
2	Central canal	11	Spinal nerve, anterior (ventral) root (ramus)
3	Posterior (dorsal) spinal artery	12	Anterior spinal artery
4	Posterior (dorsal) horn	13	Arterial vasocorona
5	Arterial vasocorona	14	Sulcal commissural arteries
6	Anterior (ventral) horn	15	Anterior funiculus
7	Spinal nerve, posterior (dorsal) root (ramus)	16	Lateral funiculus
8	Posterior (dorsal) root ganglion	17	Posterior spinal artery
9	Mixed spinal nerve		

Brain Slices

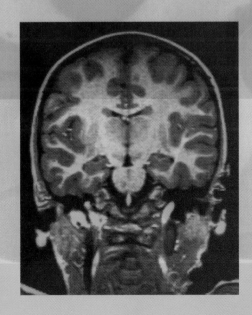

1. Coronal Sections

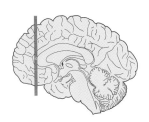

Coronal Section Through Rostral Wall of Lateral Ventricle (1X) with Vessel Territories (0.7X)

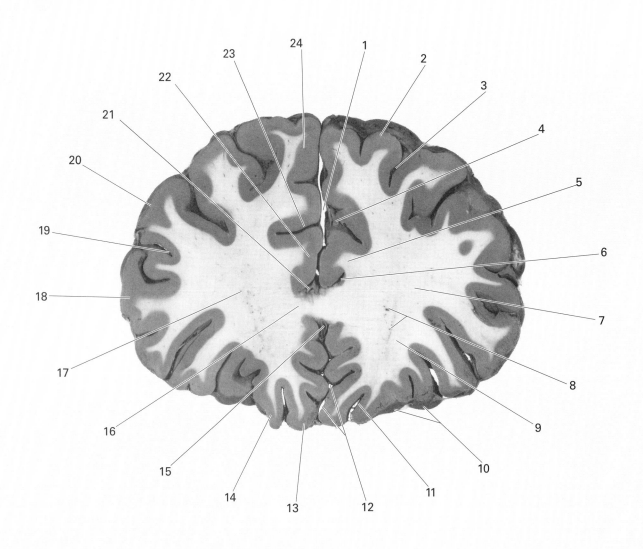

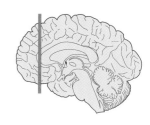

1 Longitudinal cerebral (interhemispheric) fissure
2 Superior frontal gyrus
3 Superior frontal sulcus
4 Anterior cerebral artery, callosomarginal branch
5 Cingulum
6 Callosal sulcus
7 Corpus callosum, radiations
8 Intracerebral veins
9 Inferior occipitofrontal fasciculus
10 Orbital gyri
11 Olfactory sulcus
12 Longitudinal cerebral (interhemispheric) fissure
13 Gyrus rectus (straight gyrus)
14 Medial orbital gyrus
15 Anterior cerebral artery
16 Corpus callosum, genu
17 Superior occipitofrontal fasciculus
18 Inferior frontal gyrus
19 Inferior frontal sulcus
20 Middle frontal gyrus
21 Anterior cerebral artery, pericallosal branch
22 Cingulate gyrus
23 Cingulate sulcus
24 Superior frontal gyrus
25 Anterior cerebral artery territory
26 Middle cerebral artery territory

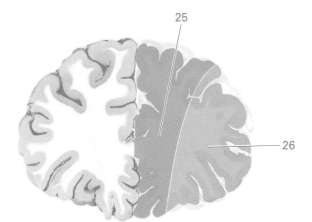

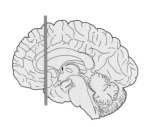

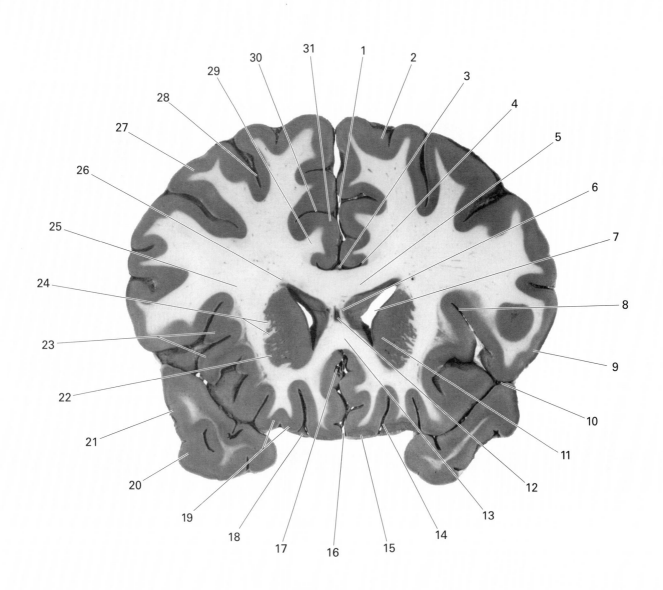

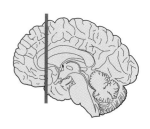

1	Longitudinal cerebral (interhemispheric) fissure
2	Superior frontal gyrus
3	Anterior cerebral artery, pericallosal branch
4	Callosal sulcus
5	Corpus callosum
6	Septum pellucidum, lamina
7	Lateral ventricle, frontal (anterior) horn
8	Circular sulcus
9	Inferior frontal gyrus
10	Lateral sulcus (*Sylvian* fissure)
11	Caudate nucleus, head
12	Septum pellucidum, cavum
13	Corpus callosum, rostrum
14	Olfactory sulcus
15	Gyrus rectus (straight gyrus)
16	Longitudinal cerebral (interhemispheric) fissure
17	Anterior cerebral artery
18	Olfactory tract
19	Orbital gyri
20	Middle temporal gyrus
21	Superior temporal gyrus
22	Putamen
23	Insula, short gyri
24	Internal capsule, anterior limb
25	Superior longitudinal fasciculus
26	Superior occipitofrontal fasciculus
27	Middle frontal gyrus
28	Superior frontal sulcus
29	Cingulum
30	Cingulate sulcus
31	Cingulate gyrus
32	Calvarium and subcutaneous fat
33	Lateral ventricle, frontal (anterior) horn
34	Temporalis muscle
35	Ethmoidal air cells
36	Orbital fat
37	Floor of anterior cranial fossa

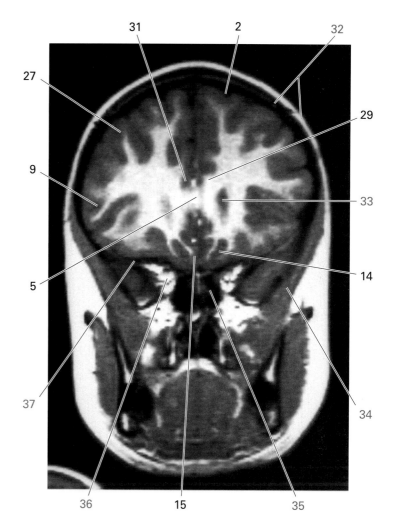

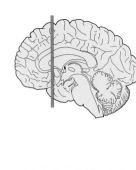

Coronal Section Through Head of Caudate Nucleus and Putamen (1X) with MRI (0.7X)

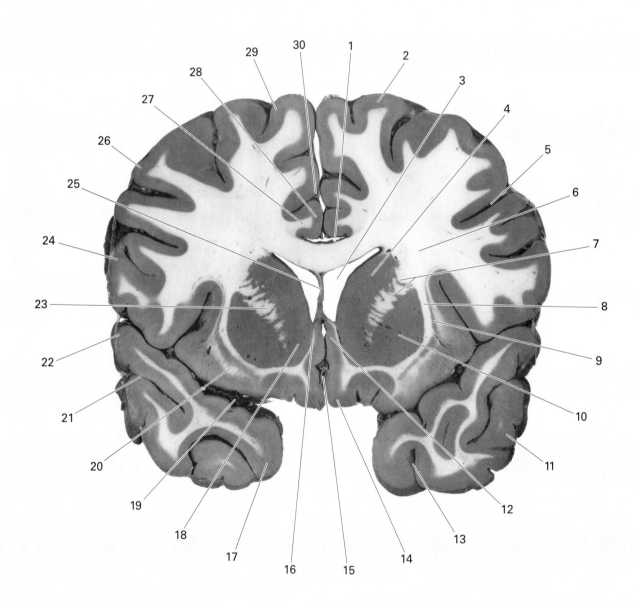

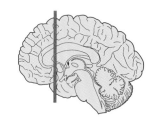

1	Callosal sulcus
2	Superior frontal gyrus
3	Lateral ventricle, frontal (anterior) horn
4	Caudate nucleus, head
5	Inferior frontal sulcus
6	Corona radiata
7	Caudatolenticular gray bridges
8	External capsule
9	Claustrum
10	Putamen
11	Middle temporal gyrus
12	Cingulate gyrus
13	Inferior temporal sulcus
14	Gyrus rectus (straight gyrus)
15	Anterior cerebral artery
16	Cingulum
17	Inferior temporal gyrus
18	Nucleus accumbens septi
19	Middle cerebral artery
20	Extreme capsule
21	Superior temporal sulcus
22	Superior temporal gyrus
23	Internal capsule, anterior limb
24	Inferior frontal gyrus
25	Septum pellucidum
26	Middle frontal gyrus
27	Cingulum
28	Cingulate gyrus
29	Superior frontal gyrus
30	Anterior cerebral artery, callosomarginal branch
31	Clivus
32	Carotid siphon

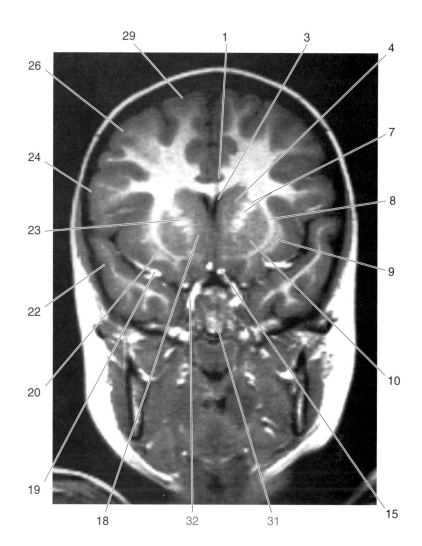

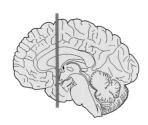

Coronal Section Through Anterior Limit of Amygdala (1X) with Vessel Territories (0.7X)

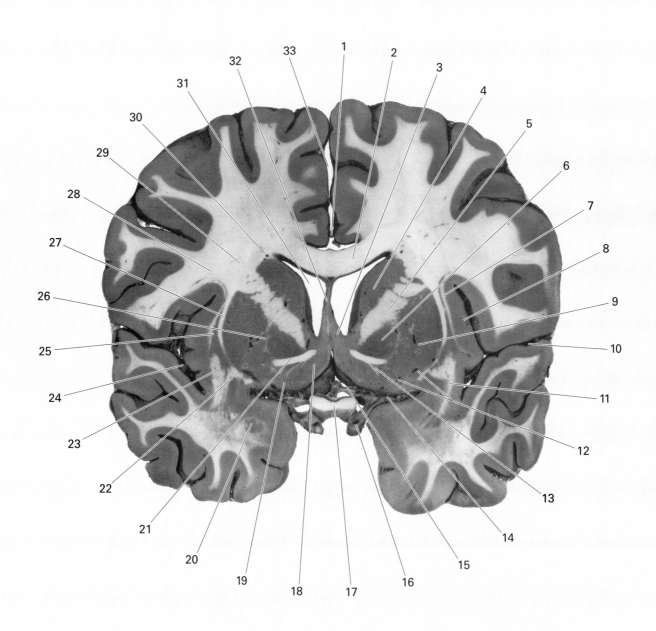

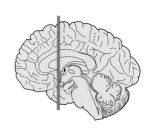

1 Anterior cerebral artery, pericallosal branch
2 Corpus callosum, body
3 Lateral septal nucleus
4 Caudate nucleus, head
5 Internal capsule, anterior limb
6 Globus pallidus, external (lateral) segment (GPe)
7 Extreme capsule
8 Insula
9 Putamen
10 Lateral sulcus (*Sylvian* fissure)
11 Uncinate fasciculus
12 Middle cerebral artery, lateral lenticulostriate branches [medial lenticulostriate branches originate from the anterior cerebral artery]
13 Anterior commissure, olfactory part
14 Middle cerebral artery
15 Anterior cerebral artery
16 Internal carotid artery
17 Optic chiasm
18 Nucleus of diagonal band (diagonal band of *Broca*)
19 Anterior perforated substance
20 Amygdala
21 Anterior commissure
22 Orbitofrontal fibers
23 Inferior occipitofrontal fasciculus
24 Middle cerebral artery
25 Claustrum
26 Globus pallidus, lateral medullary lamina
27 External capsule
28 Superior longitudinal fasciculus
29 Corona radiata
30 Superior occipitofrontal fasciculus
31 Lateral ventricle, frontal (anterior) horn
32 Septum pellucidum
33 Longitudinal cerebral (interhemispheric) fissure
34 Anterior cerebral artery territories
35 Middle cerebral artery territory
36 Choroidal arteries territory
37 Posterior cerebral artery territory

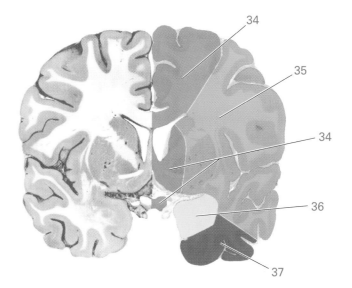

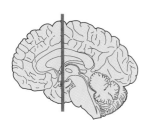

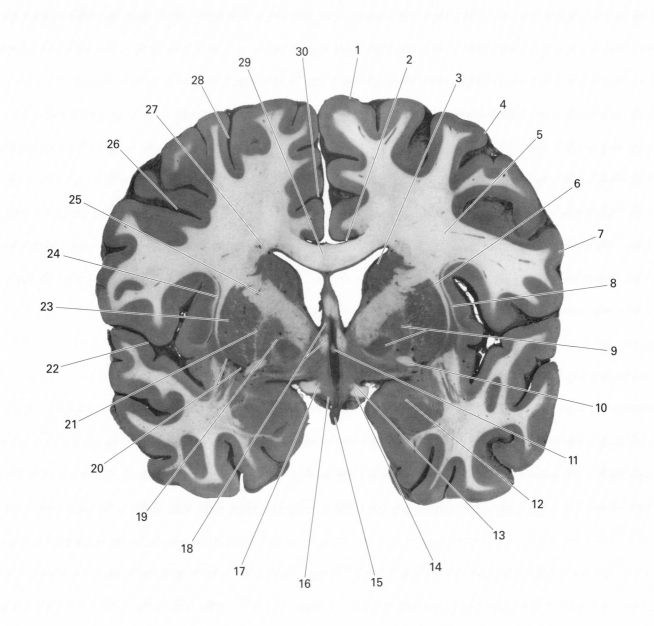

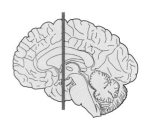

1 Superior frontal gyrus
2 Callosal sulcus
3 Caudate nucleus, head
4 Middle frontal gyrus
5 Corona radiata
6 External capsule
7 Inferior frontal gyrus
8 Extreme capsule
9 Globus pallidus, external (lateral) and internal (medial) segments (GPe and GPi)
10 Anterior commissure, descending limb
11 Anterior commissure
12 Amygdala
13 Dorsal supraoptic commissure
14 Optic tract
15 Infundibulum, pituitary stalk
16 Tuber cinereum
17 Ventral supraoptic commissure
18 Fornix, column
19 Globus pallidus, medial medullary lamina
20 Middle cerebral artery, lateral lenticulostriate branches [medial lenticulostriate branches originate from the anterior cerebral artery]
21 Globus pallidus, lateral medullary lamina
22 Lateral sulcus (*Sylvian* fissure)
23 Putamen
24 Claustrum
25 Internal capsule, anterior limb
26 Inferior frontal sulcus
27 Superior occipitofrontal fasciculus
28 Superior frontal sulcus
29 Corpus callosum, body
30 Cingulate sulcus
31 Internal carotid artery
32 Clivus
33 Middle cerebral artery stem
34 Middle cerebral artery, branches
35 Lateral ventricle

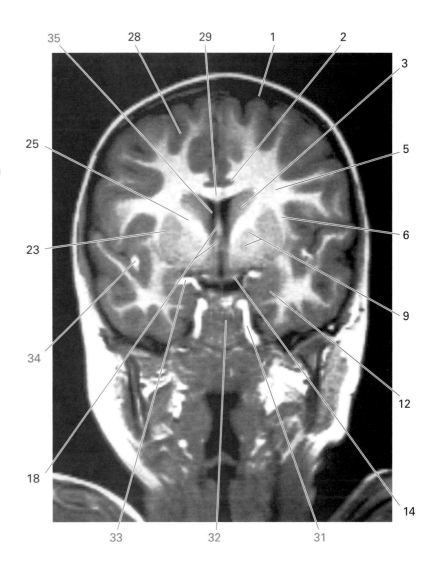

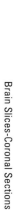

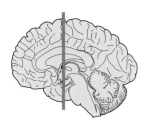

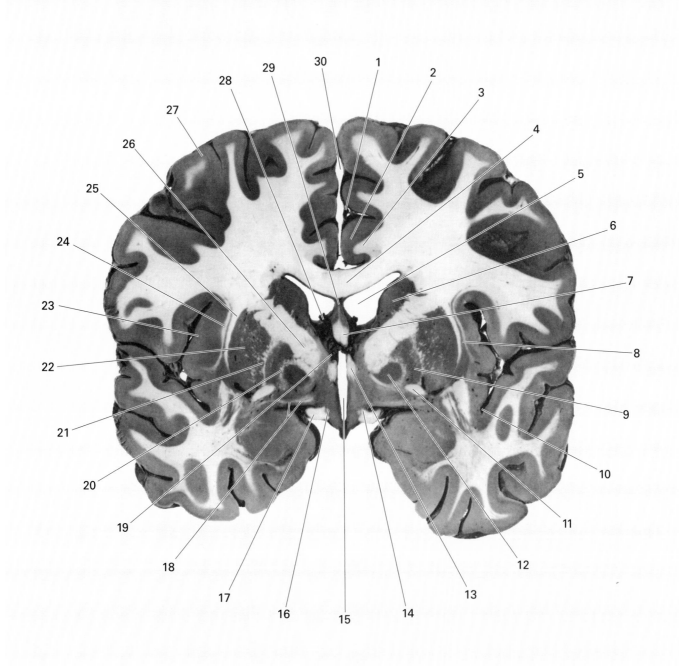

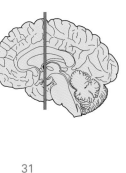

1 Anterior cerebral artery, callosomarginal branch
2 Cingulate gyrus
3 Cingulum
4 Corpus callosum, body
5 Lateral ventricle, body
6 Caudate nucleus, head
7 Fornix, body
8 Claustrum
9 Globus pallidus, external (lateral) segment (GPe)
10 Circular sulcus
11 Anterior commissure
12 Globus pallidus, internal (medial) segment (GPi)
   and underlying nucleus basalis (nucleus basalis
   of *Meynert*)
13 Fornix, column
14 Dorsal supraoptic commissure
15 Third ventricle (III)
16 Ventral supraoptic commissure
17 Optic tract
18 Ansa peduncularis
19 Interventricular foramen (foramen of *Monro*)
20 Globus pallidus, medial medullary lamina
21 Globus pallidus, lateral medullary lamina
22 Putamen
23 Insula
24 Extreme capsule
25 External capsule
26 Internal capsule, genu
27 Middle frontal gyrus
28 Choroid plexus of lateral ventricle
29 Septum pellucidum
30 Longitudinal cerebral (interhemispheric) fissure
31 Anterior cerebral artery territory
32 Middle cerebral artery territory
33 Posterior communicating artery territory
34 Posterior cerebral artery territory
35 Choroidal arteries territory
36 Internal carotid artery territory

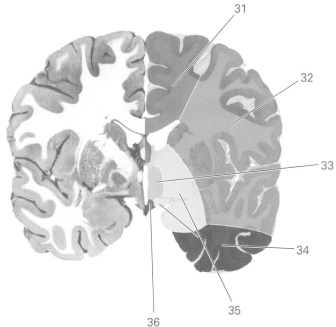

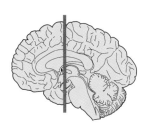

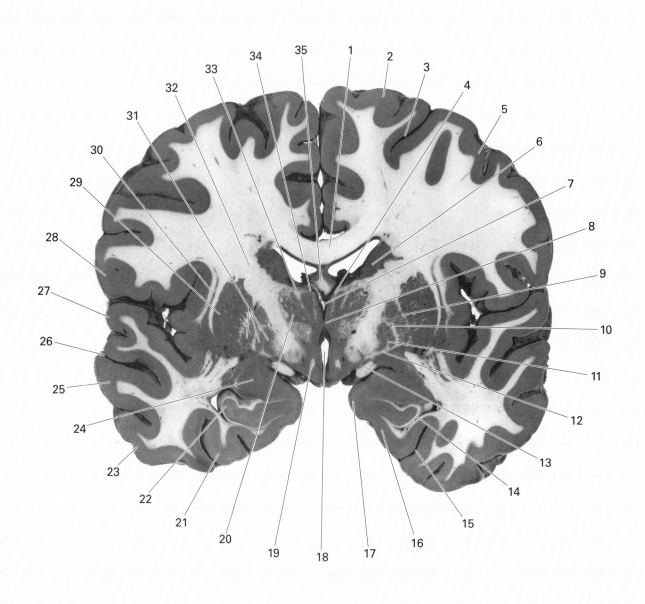

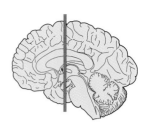

1 Corpus callosum, body
2 Superior frontal gyrus
3 Superior frontal sulcus
4 Stria medullaris of thalamus
5 Middle frontal gyrus
6 Caudate nucleus, body
7 Third ventricle (III)
8 Interthalamic adhesion (massa intermedia)
9 Globus pallidus, lateral medullary lamina
10 Globus pallidus, medial medullary lamina
11 Globus pallidus, accessory medullary lamina
12 Ansa lenticularis and nucleus basalis (nucleus basalis of *Meynert*)
13 Optic tract
14 Hippocampus, alveus
15 Collateral sulcus
16 Parahippocampal gyrus
17 Uncus
18 Third ventricle (III)
19 Fornix, column
20 Thalamus, ventral anterior nucleus (VA)
21 Lateral occipitotemporal (fusiform) gyrus
22 Hippocampus
23 Inferior temporal gyrus
24 Amygdala
25 Middle temporal gyrus
26 Superior temporal sulcus
27 Superior temporal gyrus
28 Inferior frontal gyrus
29 Putamen
30 Claustrum
31 Globus pallidus, external (lateral) and internal (medial) segments (GPe and GPi)
32 Internal capsule, posterior limb
33 Thalamus, internal medullary lamina
34 Thalamus, anterior nucleus (A)
35 Fornix, body
36 Posterior cerebral artery
37 Internal carotid artery, intrapetrous part
38 Clivus
39 Lateral ventricle, temporal (inferior) horn

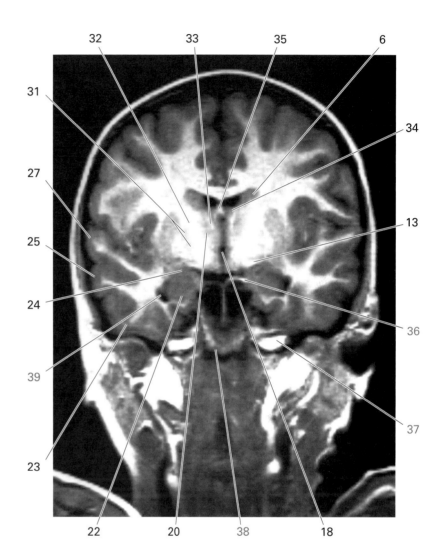

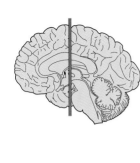

Coronal Section Through Mamillothalamic Tract (Fasciculus) (1X) with Vessel Territories (0.7X)

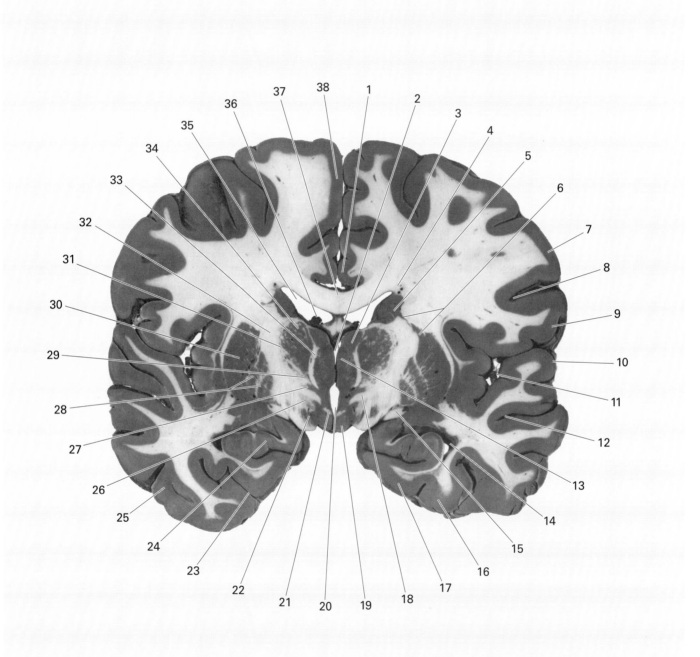

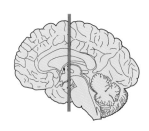

1   Cingulate gyrus
2   Third ventricle (III)
3   Thalamus, anterior nucleus (A)
4   Superior occipitofrontal fasciculus
5   Caudate nucleus, tail
6   Caudatolenticular gray matter striae
7   Precentral gyrus
8   Central sulcus (fissure of *Rolando*)
9   Postcentral gyrus
10 Superior temporal gyrus
11 Middle cerebral artery
12 Superior temporal sulcus
13 Thalamus, dorsomedial nucleus (DM)
14 Lateral ventricle, temporal (inferior) horn
15 Optic tract
16 Lateral occipitotemporal gyrus
17 Parahippocampal gyrus
18 Lenticular fasciculus (H2 field of *Forel*)
19 Mamillary body
20 Third ventricle (III)
21 Principal mamillary fasciculus
22 Substantia nigra
23 Collateral sulcus
24 Dentate gyrus
25 Inferior temporal gyrus
26 Subthalamic nucleus
27 Zona incerta
28 Globus pallidus, external (lateral) and internal (medial)
    segments (GPe and GPi)
29 Thalamic fasciculus (H1 field of *Forel*)
30 Putamen
31 Thalamus, external medullary lamina
32 Internal capsule, posterior limb
33 Mamillothalamic tract
34 Thalamus, lateroposterior nucleus (LP)
35 Lateral ventricle, body
36 Choroid plexus of lateral ventricle
37 Corpus callosum, body
38 Superior frontal gyrus
39 Anterior cerebral artery territory
40 Middle cerebral artery territory
41 Choroidal arteries territory
42 Posterior cerebral artery territory
43 Posterior communicating artery territory

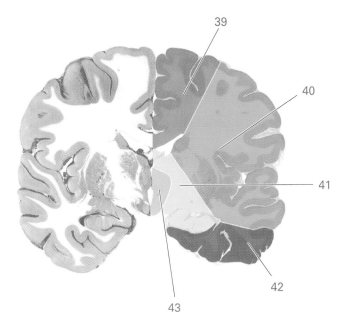

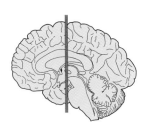

Coronal Section Through Mamillary Bodies (1X) with MRI (0.7X)

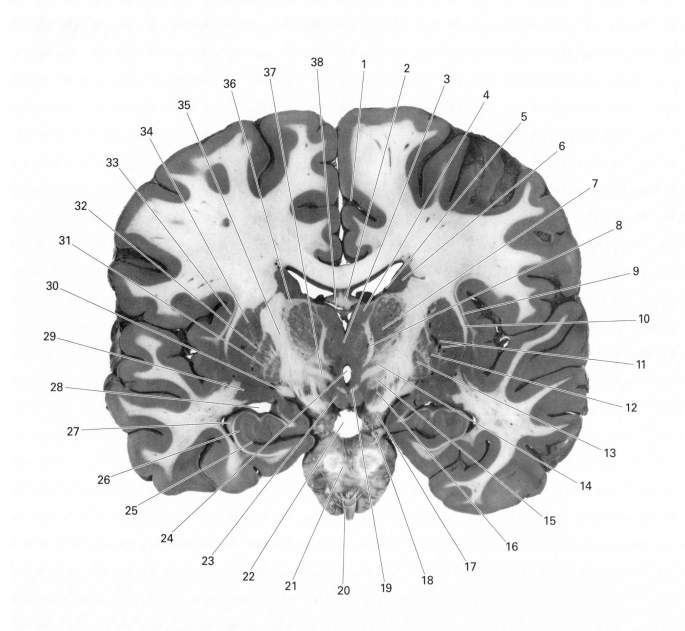

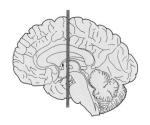

1	Anterior cerebral artery, callosomarginal branch
2	Fornix, body
3	Interthalamic adhesion (massa intermedia, interthalamic connexus)
4	Thalamus, anterior nucleus (A)
5	Stria terminalis and thalamostriate vein
6	Caudate nucleus, tail
7	Thalamus, ventral lateral nucleus (VL)
8	Mamillothalamic tract
9	Claustrum
10	External capsule
11	Middle cerebral artery, lateral lenticulostriate branches [medial lenticulostriate branches originate from the anterior cerebral artery]
12	Globus pallidus, internal (medial) segments (GPi)
13	Globus pallidus, external (lateral) segments (GPe)
14	Zona incerta
15	Subthalamic nucleus
16	Substantia nigra
17	Cerebral peduncle
18	Posterior cerebral artery
19	Principal mamillary fasciculus
20	Basilar artery
21	Pons
22	Interpeduncular fossa
23	Mamillary body
24	Third ventricle (III)
25	Uncal fissure
26	Hippocampus
27	Hippocampus, alveus
28	Lateral ventricle, temporal (inferior) horn
29	Amygdala and nucleus basalis (nucleus basalis of *Meynert*)
30	Optic tract
31	Globus pallidus, medial medullary lamina
32	Globus pallidus, lateral medullary lamina
33	Extreme capsule
34	Putamen
35	Internal capsule, posterior limb
36	Thalamus, rostral peduncle
37	Lenticular fasciculus (H2 field of *Forel*)
38	Velum interpositum
39	Lateral ventricle, body
40	Lateral sulcus (*Sylvian* fissure)

41	Internal carotid artery
42	Cerebral peduncle
43	External capsule

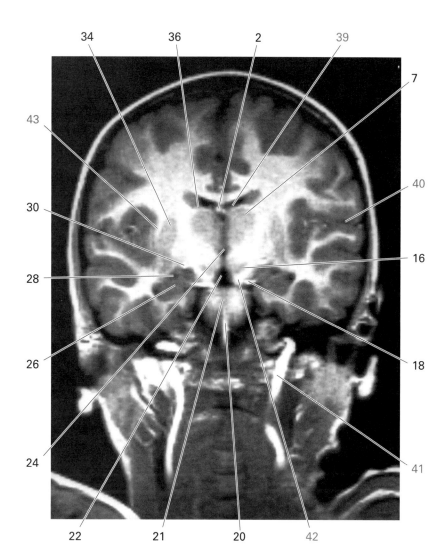

Brain Slices-Coronal Sections

65

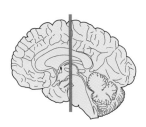

Coronal Section Through Subthalamic Nucleus (1X) with Vessel Territories (0.7X)

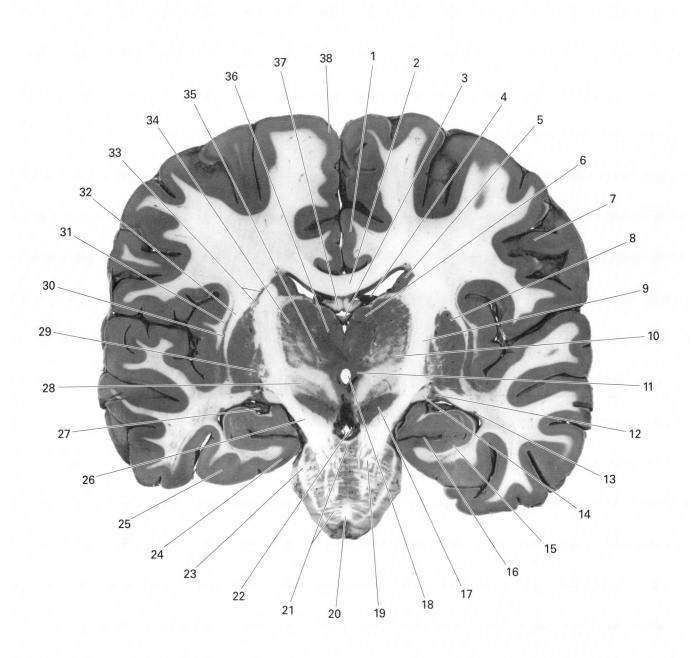

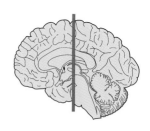

1 Cingulate gyrus
2 Corpus callosum, body
3 Velum interpositum and tela choroidea
4 Choroid plexus of lateral ventricle
5 Caudate nucleus, tail
6 Thalamus, anterior nucleus (A)
7 Postcentral gyrus
8 Putamen
9 Internal capsule, posterior limb
10 Thalamus, ventral posterolateral nucleus (VPL)
11 Hypothalamus
12 Amygdala
13 Caudate nucleus, tail
14 Optic tract
15 Hippocampus
16 Uncal fissure
17 Substantia nigra
18 Third ventricle (III)
19 Corticospinal (pyramidal) tract
20 Ventral decussation of pons
21 Superficial transverse fibers of pons
22 Interpeduncular fossa
23 Middle cerebellar peduncle (brachium pontis)
24 Parahippocampal gyrus
25 Lateral occipitotemporal gyrus
26 Cerebral peduncle
27 Choroid plexus of lateral ventricle, temporal (inferior) horn
28 Subthalamic nucleus
29 Globus pallidus, external (lateral) segment (GPe)
30 Claustrum
31 Extreme capsule
32 External capsule
33 Caudatolenticular gray matter striae
34 Thalamus, lateroposterior nucleus (LP)
35 Thalamus, internal medullary lamina
36 Thalamus, dorsomedial nucleus (DM)
37 Fornix, body
38 Superior frontal gyrus
39 Anterior cerebral artery territory
40 Middle cerebral artery territory
41 Choroidal arteries territory
42 Posterior cerebral artery territory
43 Posterior cerebral artery, perforating branches territory
44 Basilar artery, lateral branches territory
45 Basilar artery, medial branches territory

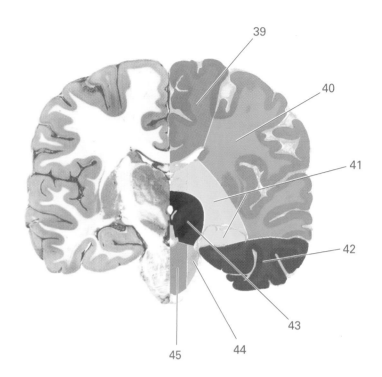

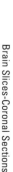

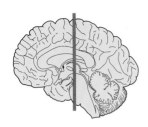

Coronal Section Through Posterior Limit of Interpeduncular Fossa (1X) with MRI (0.7X)

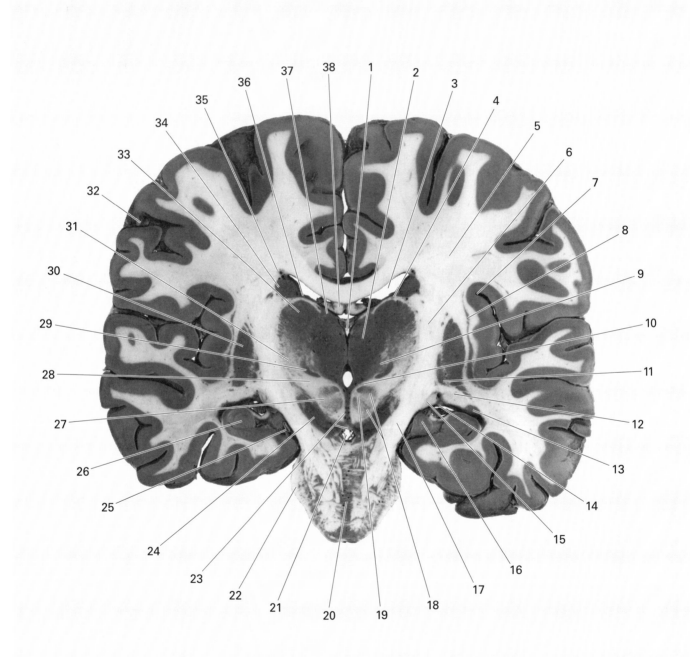

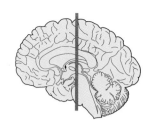

1	Third ventricle (III)
2	Thalamus, dorsomedial nucleus (DM)
3	Lateral ventricle, body
4	Thalamus, rostral peduncle
5	Corona radiata
6	Internal capsule, posterior limb
7	Circular sulcus
8	Claustrum
9	Thalamus, centromedian nucleus (CM)
10	Medial longitudinal fasciculus
11	Globus pallidus, external (lateral) segment (GPe)
12	Optic radiation
13	Caudate nucleus, tail
14	Stria terminalis
15	Optic tract
16	Uncus
17	Cerebral peduncle
18	Red nucleus
19	Habenulo-interpeduncular tract (fasciculus retroflexus of *Meynert*)
20	Pons
21	Interpeduncular fossa
22	Middle cerebellar peduncle
23	Interpeduncular nucleus
24	Substantia nigra
25	Posterior cerebral artery
26	Hippocampus
27	Red nucleus, medullary lamina
28	Medial lemniscus
29	Thalamus, ventroposteromedial nucleus (VPM)
30	Putamen
31	Thalamus, ventroposterolateral nucleus (VPL)
32	Central sulcus (fissure of *Rolando*)
33	Thalamus, lateroposterior nucleus (LP)
34	Caudate nucleus, tail
35	Superior occipitofrontal fasciculus
36	Stria terminalis
37	Thalamus, laterodorsal nucleus (LD)
38	Fornix, body
39	Hippocampus, alveus
40	Inferior temporal gyrus
41	Apex of petrous bone
42	Basilar artery
43	Occipitotemporal sulcus
44	Optic tract
45	Claustrum

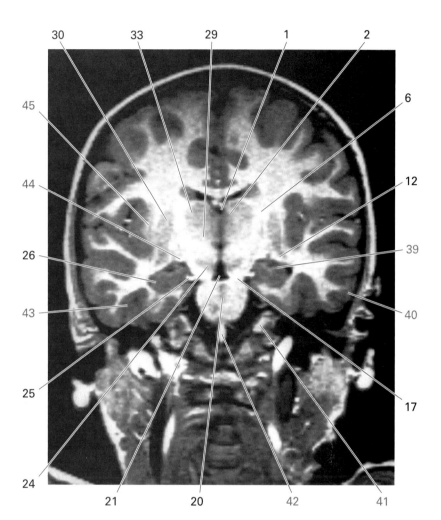

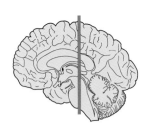

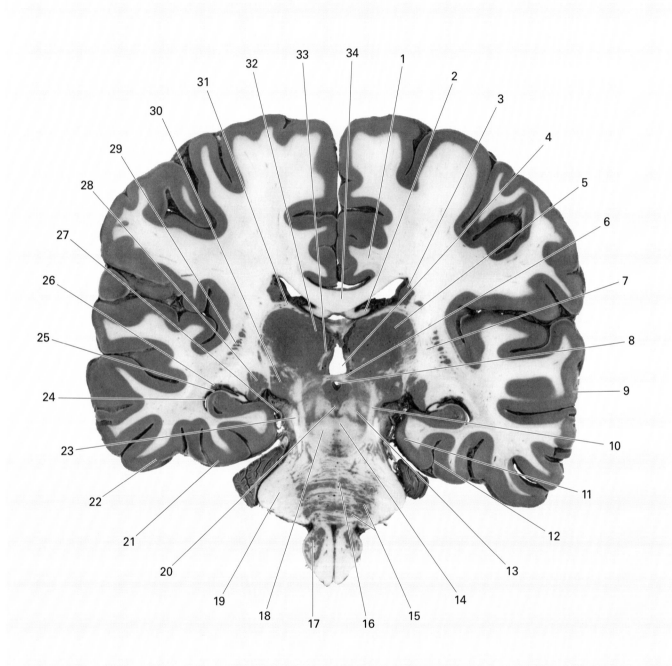

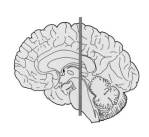

1 Cingulum
2 Fornix, crus
3 Caudate nucleus, tail
4 Third ventricle (III)
5 Thalamus, lateroposterior nucleus (LP)
6 Posterior commissure
7 Internal capsule, posterior limb
8 Cerebral aqueduct (aqueduct of *Sylvius*)
9 Superior temporal gyrus
10 Medial lemniscus
11 Parahippocampal gyrus
12 Collateral sulcus
13 Central tegmental tract
14 Superior cerebellar peduncle, decussations
15 Pontine nuclei
16 Raphé of pons
17 Inferior olivary nucleus
18 Superior cerebellar peduncle (brachium conjunctivum)
19 Middle cerebellar peduncle (brachium pontis)
20 Medial longitudinal fasciculus
21 Lateral occipitotemporal gyrus
22 Inferior temporal gyrus
23 Lateral lemniscus
24 Lateral ventricle, temporal (inferior) horn
25 Hippocampus, alveus
26 Caudate nucleus, tail
27 Posterior cerebral artery
28 Thalamus, lateral geniculate nucleus (LGN)
   (lateral geniculate body)
29 Transcapsular caudatolenticular gray striae
30 Thalamus, medial geniculate nucleus (MG)
   (medial geniculate body)
31 Thalamus, rostral peduncle
32 Thalamus, dorsomedial nucleus (DM)
33 Habenulo-interpeduncular tract (fasciculus retroflexus
   of *Meynert*)
34 Corpus callosum, body
35 Anterior cerebral artery territory
36 Middle cerebral artery territory
37 Choroidal arteries territory
38 Posterior cerebral artery, collicular and posterior
   choroidal branches territory
39 Posterior cerebral artery, perforating branches territory
40 Posterior cerebral artery territory
41 Superior cerebellar artery territory
42 Anterior inferior cerebellar artery territory
43 Basilar artery, lateral branches territory
44 Basilar artery, medial branches territory
45 Posterior inferior cerebellar artery territory
46 Vertebral artery territory
47 Anterior spinal artery territory

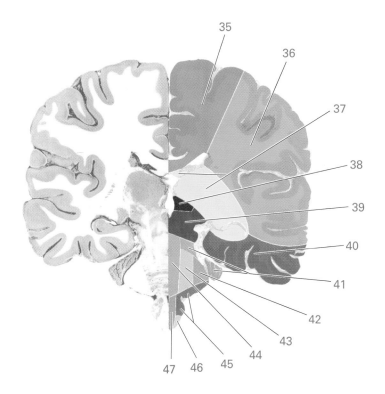

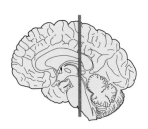

Coronal Section Through Commissure of Superior Colliculi (1X) with MRI (0.7X)

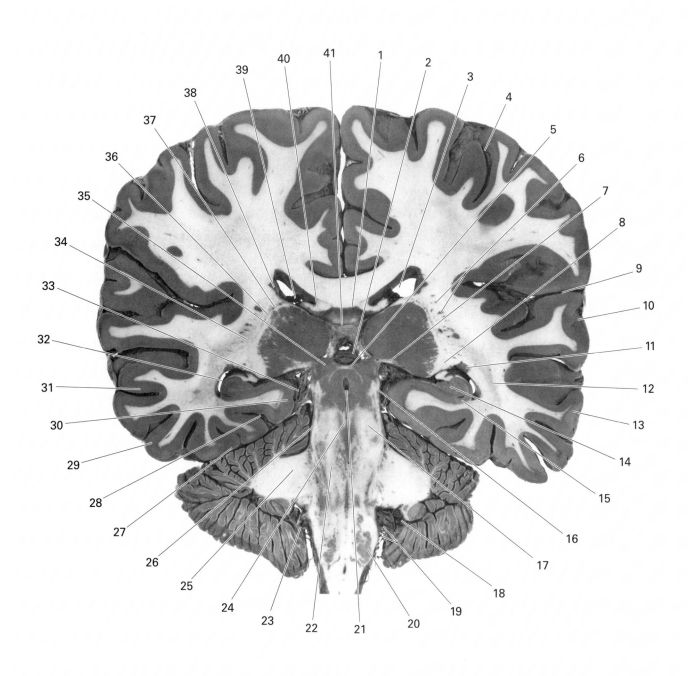

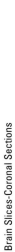

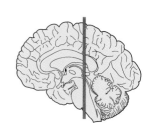

1	Fornix, commissure
2	Pineal gland
3	Lateral ventricle, body
4	Central sulcus (fissure of *Rolando*)
5	Commissure of superior colliculus
6	Caudatolenticular gray matter striae
7	Superior colliculus, brachium
8	Triangular area
9	Lateral sulcus (*Sylvian* fissure)
10	Superior temporal gyrus
11	Caudate nucleus, tail
12	Optic radiation
13	Middle temporal gyrus
14	Dentate gyrus
15	Hippocampus
16	Inferior colliculus, brachium
17	Superior cerebellar peduncle (brachium conjunctivum)
18	Lateral recess of fourth ventricle (IV)
19	Vagus nerve, rootlets (CN X)
20	Inferior olivary nucleus
21	Cerebral aqueduct (aqueduct of *Sylvius*)
22	Central tegmental fasciculus
23	Glossopharyngeal nerve (CN IX)
24	Medial longitudinal fasciculus
25	Middle cerebellar peduncle (brachium pontis)
26	Lateral lemniscus
27	Lateral occipitotemporal gyrus
28	Collateral sulcus
29	Inferior temporal gyrus
30	Parahippocampal gyrus
31	Middle temporal gyrus
32	Lateral ventricle, temporal (inferior) horn
33	Posterior cerebral artery
34	Internal capsule, posterior limb
35	Superior colliculus
36	Thalamus, external medullary lamina
37	Thalamus, reticular nucleus
38	Caudate nucleus, tail
39	Choroid plexus of lateral ventrical
40	Fornix, crus
41	Velum interpositum
42	Cerebellar hemisphere
43	Occipital condyle
44	Lateral mass of atlas
45	Medulla oblongata

46	Vertebral artery
47	Hippocampus, fimbria

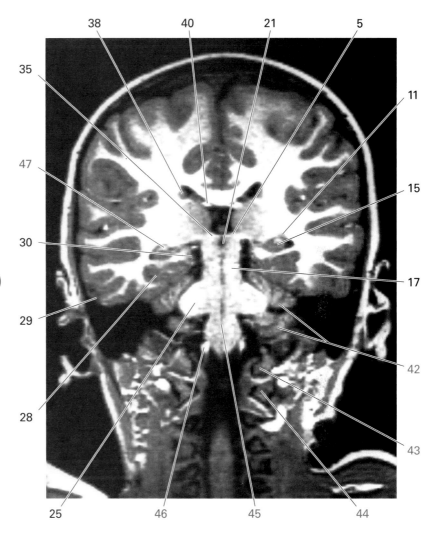

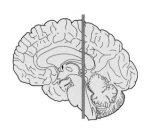

Coronal Section Through Quadrigeminal Plate (1X) with Vessel Territories (0.7X)

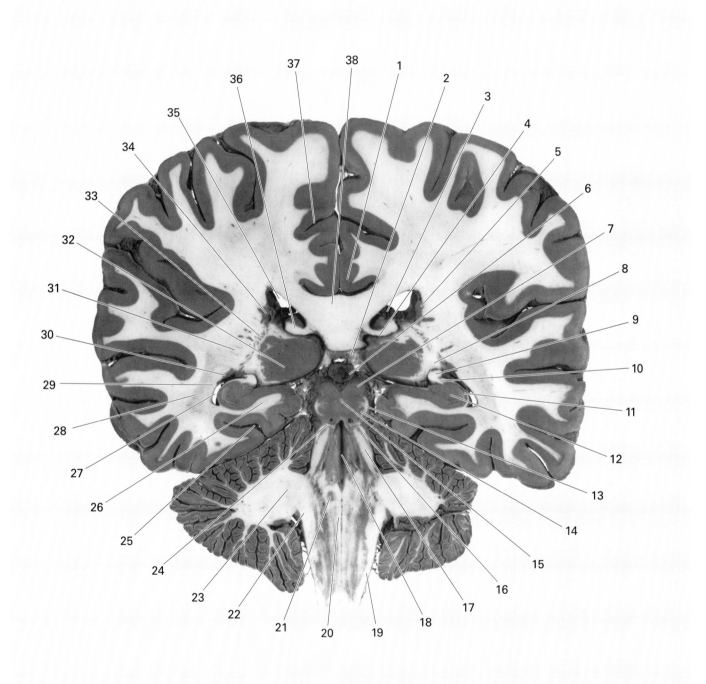

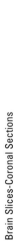

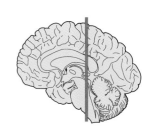

1 Cingulate gyrus
2 Internal cerebral vein
3 Choroid plexus of lateral ventricle
4 Choroidal fissure
5 Caudate nucleus, tail
6 Pineal gland
7 Superior colliculus
8 Triangular area
9 Hippocampus, fimbria
10 Hippocampus, alveus
11 Hippocampus (*Sommer's* sector)
12 Dentate gyrus
13 Inferior colliculus, brachium
14 Inferior colliculus
15 Commissure of inferior colliculus
16 Uncinate fasciculus
17 Superior cerebellar peduncle (brachium conjunctivum)
18 Median sulcus of fourth ventricle (IV)
19 Posterior (dorsal) spinocerebellar tract
20 Medial longitudinal fasciculus
21 Abducent nucleus (CN VI)
22 Inferior cerebellar peduncle (restiform body)
23 Middle cerebellar peduncle (brachium pontis)
24 Trochlear nerve (IV)
25 Collateral sulcus
26 Cingulum
27 Lateral ventricle, temporal (inferior) horn
28 Optic radiation
29 Tapetum
30 Caudate nucleus, tail
31 Internal capsule, retrolenticular part
32 Thalamus, pulvinar (Pul)
33 Caudatolenticular gray matter striae
34 Thalamostriate vein
35 Lateral ventricle, body
36 Fornix, crus
37 Cingulate sulcus
38 Corpus callosum, splenium

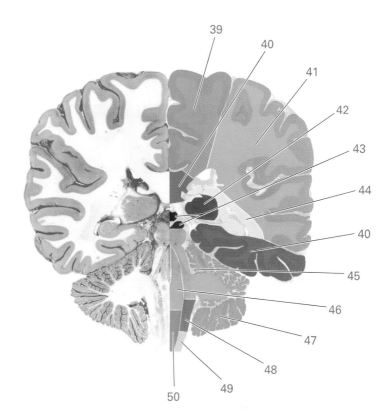

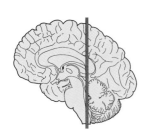

Coronal Section Through Fourth Ventricle (IV) (1X) with MRI (0.7X)

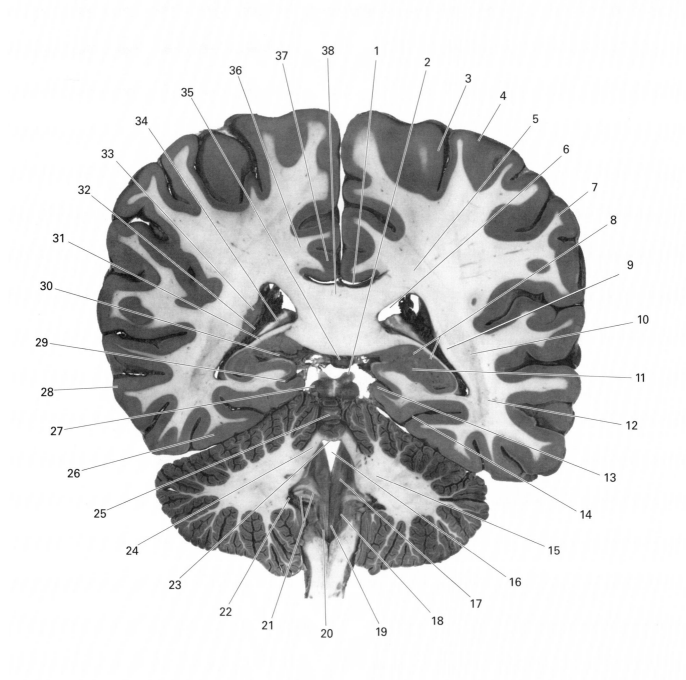

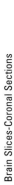

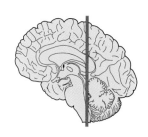

1 Callosal sulcus
2 Superior colliculus
3 Precentral gyrus
4 Postcentral gyrus
5 Corpus callosum, forceps major
6 Lateral ventricle, trigone (atrium)
7 Inferior parietal lobule
8 Retrosplenial gyri
9 Tapetum
10 Optic radiation
11 Hippocampus
12 Inferior longitudinal fasciculus
13 Medial occipitotemporal (lingual) gyrus
14 Collateral sulcus
15 Middle cerebellar peduncle (brachium pontis)
16 Fourth ventricle (IV)
17 Facial colliculus
18 Sulcus limitans
19 Hypoglossal (CN XII) trigone
20 Vagal (CN X) trigone
21 Medullary striae of fourth ventricle (IV)
22 Fourth ventricle (IV), lateral recess
23 Superior medullary velum
24 Superior cerebellar peduncle (brachium conjunctivum)
25 Cerebellum, vermis, central lobule
26 Lateral occipitotemporal gyrus
27 Inferior colliculus
28 Middle temporal gyrus
29 Calcarine fissure
30 Hippocampal sulcus
31 Hippocampus, fimbria
32 Choroid plexus of lateral ventricle
33 Caudate nucleus, tail
34 Fornix, crus
35 Pineal gland
36 Cingulum
37 Cingulate gyrus
38 Corpus callosum, splenium
39 Quadrigeminal cistern
40 Spinal cord
41 Medulla oblongata
42 Junction of hippocampus, fimbria, and fornix, crus

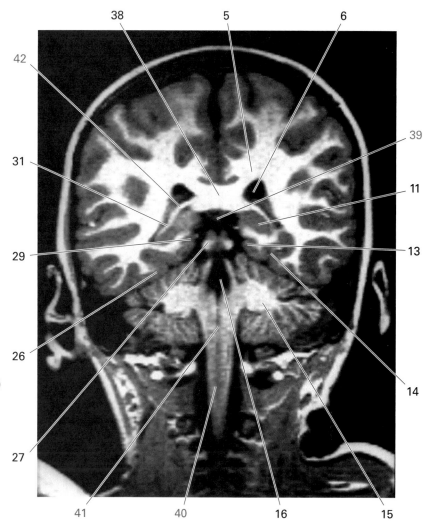

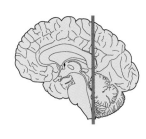

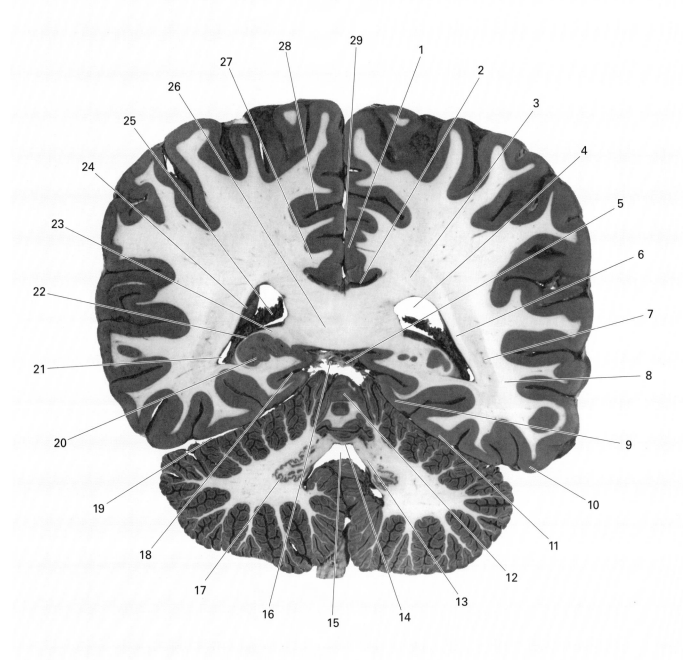

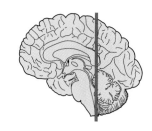

1. Cingulate gyrus
2. Indusium griseum
3. Corpus callosum, forceps major
4. Lateral ventricle, trigone (atrium)
5. Arachnoid membrane
6. Tapetum
7. Optic radiation
8. Inferior longitudinal fasciculus
9. Medial occipitotemporal (lingual) gyrus
10. Inferior temporal gyrus
11. Lateral occipitotemporal gyrus
12. Cerebellum, anterior vermis
13. Superior cerebellar peduncle (brachium conjunctivum)
14. Superior medullary velum
15. Fourth ventricle (IV)
16. Internal cerebral vein
17. Dentate nucleus
18. Calcarine fissure
19. Cerebrocerebellar fissure (transverse cerebral fissure)
20. Hippocampus
21. Lateral ventricle, temporal (inferior) horn
22. Hippocampus, alveus
23. Hippocampus, fimbria
24. Caudate nucleus, tail
25. Choroid plexus of lateral ventricle
26. Corpus callosum, splenium
27. Cingulum
28. Cingulate sulcus
29. Longitudinal cerebral (interhemispheric) fissure
30. Anterior cerebral artery territory
31. Middle cerebral artery territory
32. Choroidal arteries territory
33. Posterior cerebral artery territory
34. Superior cerebellar artery territory
35. Anterior inferior cerebellar artery territory
36. Posterior inferior cerebellar artery territory
37. Posterior spinal artery territory

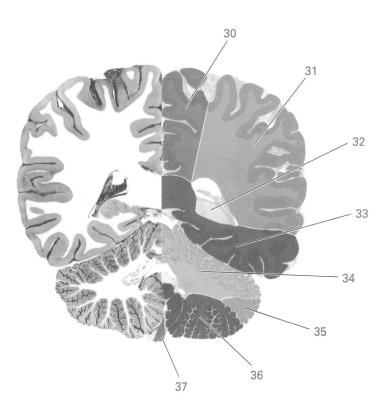

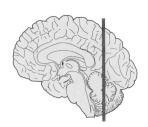

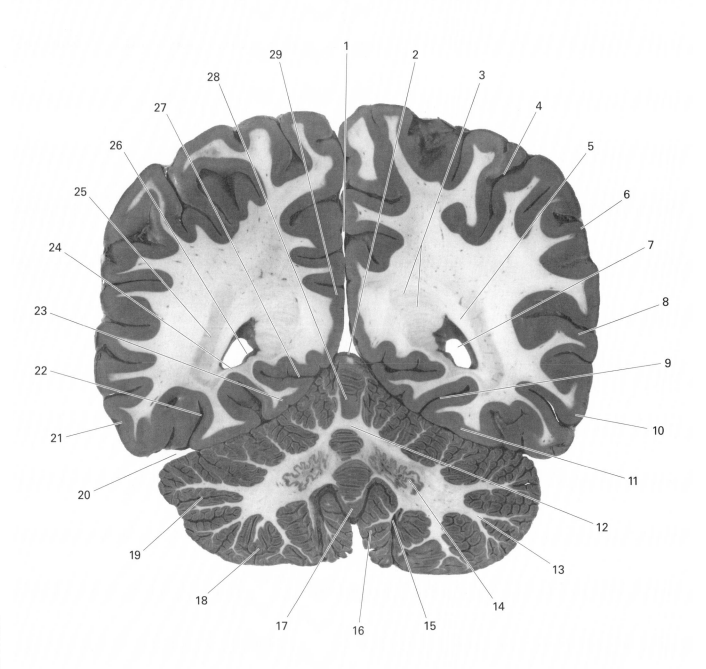

1	Longitudinal cerebral (interhemispheric) fissure
2	Cerebellum, vermis, declive
3	Corpus callosum, forceps major
4	Intraparietal sulcus
5	Tapetum
6	Inferior parietal gyrus
7	Lateral ventricle, occipital (posterior) horn
8	Superior temporal gyrus
9	Collateral sulcus
10	Middle temporal gyrus
11	Lateral occipitotemporal gyrus
12	Cerebellum, commissure
13	Cerebellum, white matter
14	Dentate nucleus
15	Secondary fissure
16	Cerebellum, tonsil
17	Cerebellum, vermis, uvula
18	Cerebellum, cortex
19	Horizontal fissure
20	Cerebrocerebellar fissure (transverse cerebral fissure)
21	Inferior temporal gyrus
22	Occipitotemporal sulcus
23	Medial occipitotemporal (lingual) gyrus
24	Collateral eminence
25	Optic radiation
26	Calcar avis (calcarine spur)
27	Calcarine fissure
28	Cerebellum, vermis, culmen
29	Precuneus
30	Foramen magnum, posterior rim
31	First cervical (C1) vertebra (atlas), posterior arch
32	Fourth ventricle (IV), posterior superior recesses

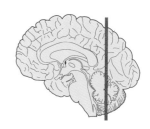

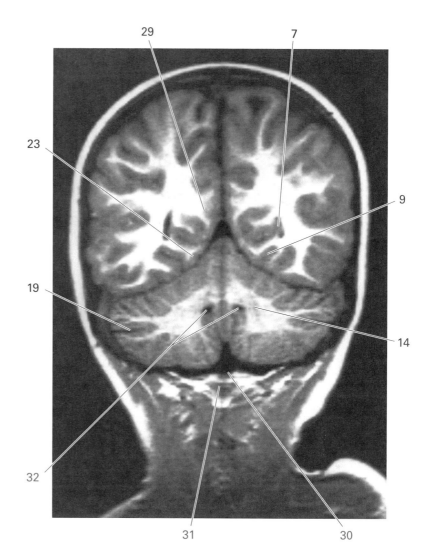

Brain Slices

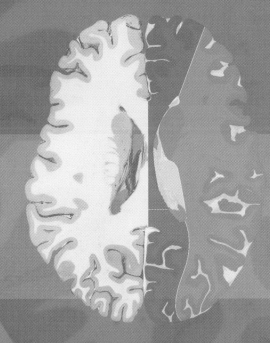

2. Axial Sections

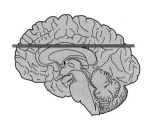

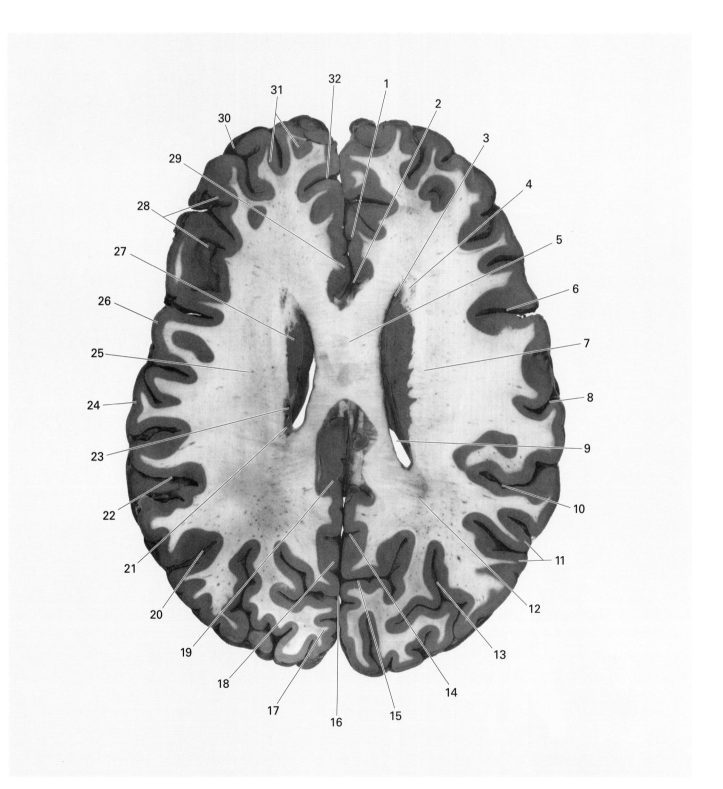

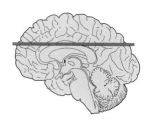

1	Cingulate gyrus
2	Anterior cerebral artery, pericallosal branch
3	Lateral ventricle, frontal (anterior) horn
4	Superior occipitofrontal fasciculus
5	Corpus callosum, body
6	Precentral sulcus
7	Corona radiata
8	Central sulcus (fissure of *Rolando*)
9	Lateral ventricle, trigone (atrium)
10	Lateral sulcus (*Sylvian* fissure)
11	Angular gyrus
12	Corpus callosum, radiations
13	Intraparietal sulcus
14	Cingulate sulcus
15	Parieto-occipital sulcus
16	Longitudinal cerebral (interhemispheric) fissure
17	Occipital lobe, cuneus
18	Medial parietal gyrus
19	Cingulate gyrus
20	Superior temporal sulcus
21	Caudate nucleus, tail
22	Lateral sulcus (*Sylvian* fissure)
23	Thalamostriate vein
24	Postcentral gyrus
25	Superior longitudinal fasciculus
26	Precentral gyrus
27	Caudate nucleus, head
28	Middle frontal gyrus
29	Cingulate gyrus
30	Superior frontal sulcus
31	Superior frontal gyrus
32	Cingulate sulcus
33	Calvarium
34	Subcutaneous fat

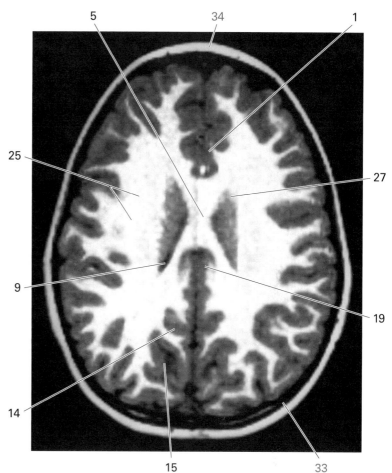

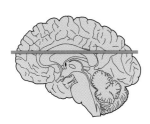

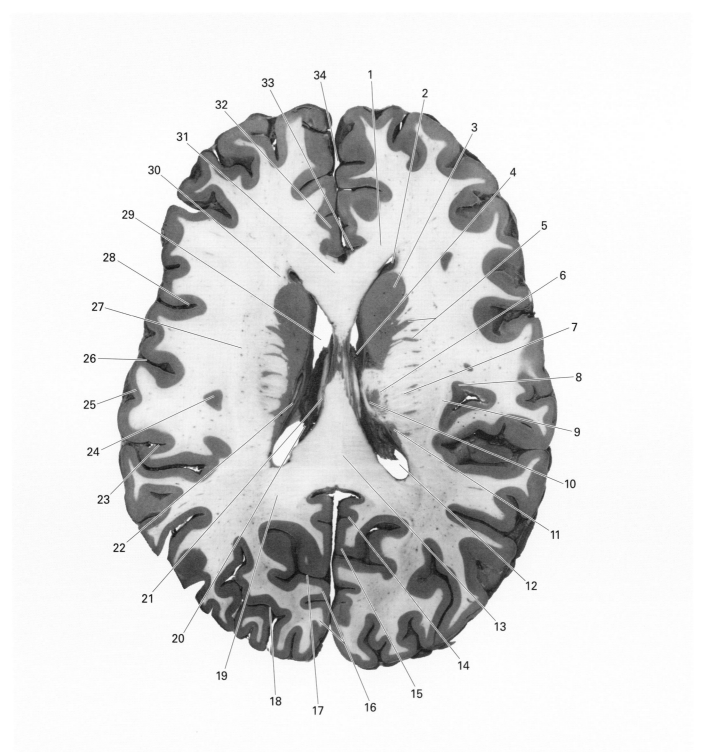

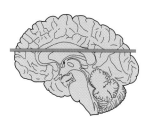

1 Corpus callosum, forceps minor
2 Lateral ventricle, frontal (anterior) horn
3 Caudate nucleus, head
4 Choroid plexus of lateral ventricle
5 Caudatolenticular gray bridges
6 Thalamus, lateroposterior nucleus (LP)
7 Internal capsule, posterior limb
8 Insula
9 Superior longitudinal fasciculus
10 Thalamus, stratum zonale
11 Caudate nucleus, tail
12 Lateral ventricle, trigone (atrium)
13 Corpus callosum, splenium
14 Cingulate sulcus
15 Parietal lobe, precuneus
16 Occipital lobe, cuneus
17 Parieto-occipital sulcus
18 Intraparietal sulcus
19 Corpus callosum, forceps major
20 Choroidal vein
21 Fornix, crus
22 Thalamostriate vein
23 Lateral sulcus (*Sylvian* fissure)
24 Insula
25 Postcentral gyrus
26 Central sulcus (fissure of *Rolando*)
27 Corona radiata
28 Precentral sulcus
29 Lateral ventricle, body
30 Superior occipitofronal fasciculus
31 Corpus callosum, genu
32 Cingulate gyrus
33 Indusium griseum
34 Longitudinal cerebral (interhemispheric) fissure
35 Anterior cerebral artery territory
36 Choroidal arteries territory
37 Middle cerebral artery territory
38 Posterior cerebral artery territory

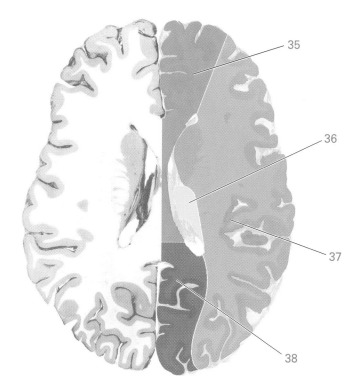

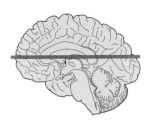

Axial Section Through Superior Putamen (1X) with MRI (0.7X)

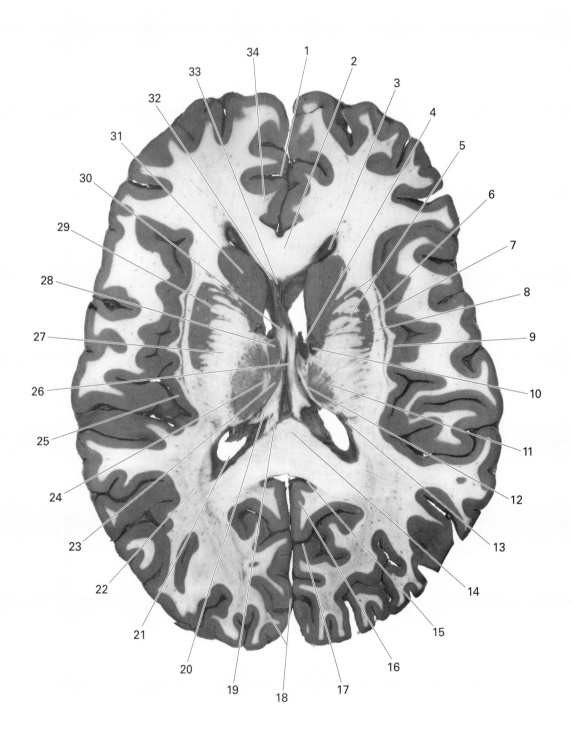

1	Cingulate sulcus
2	Corpus callosum, genu
3	Lateral ventricle, frontal (anterior) horn
4	Choroid plexus
5	Caudatolenticular gray bridges
6	Putamen
7	Extreme capsule
8	External capsule
9	Claustrum
10	Thalamostriate vein
11	Thalamus, lateroposterior nucleus (LP)
12	Thalamus, stratum zonale
13	Caudate nucleus, tail
14	Corpus callosum, splenium
15	Callosal sulcus
16	Cingulate gyrus
17	Junction of parieto-occipital sulcus and calcarine fissure
18	Occipital lobe, cuneus
19	Fornix, crus
20	Hippocampus, fimbria
21	Lateral ventricle, trigone (atrium)
22	Optic radiation
23	Thalamus, laterodorsal nucleus (LD)
24	Thalamus, internal medullary lamina
25	Insula
26	Fornix, body
27	Internal capsule, posterior limb
28	Thalamus, anterior nucleus (A)
29	Internal capsule, anterior limb
30	Fornix, body
31	Caudate nucleus, head
32	Septum pellucidum, lamina
33	Septum pellucidum, cavum
34	Cingulum
35	Junction of hippocampus, fimbria, and fornix, crus
36	Subcutaneous fat
37	Calvarium
38	Superior sagittal sinus

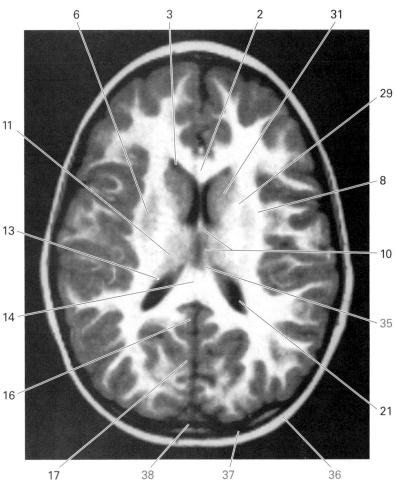

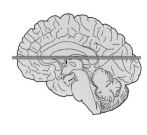

Axial Section Through Putamen (1X) with Vessel Territories (0.7X)

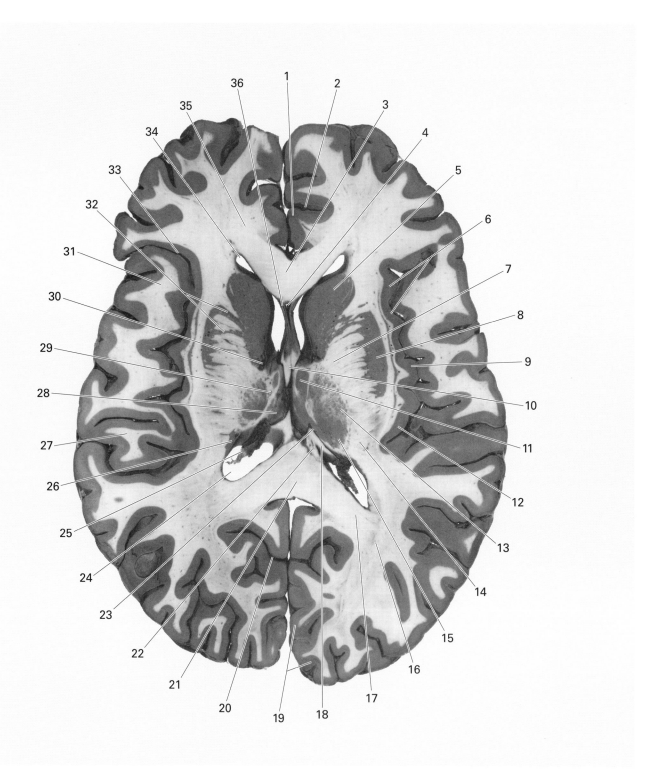

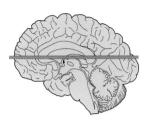

1	Cingulate gyrus
2	Cingulate sulcus
3	Corpus callosum, genu
4	Septum pellucidum, cavum
5	Caudate nucleus, head
6	Insula, short gyri
7	Internal capsule, genu
8	Putamen
9	Precentral gyrus of insula
10	Fornix, body
11	Thalamus, anterior nucleus (A)
12	Insula, long gyrus
13	Thalamus, lateroposterior nucleus (LP)
14	Internal capsule, posterior limb
15	Thalamus, pulvinar (Pul)
16	Optic radiation
17	Corpus callosum, forceps major
18	Hippocampus, fimbria
19	Occipital lobe, cuneus
20	Junction of parieto-occipital sulcus and calcarine fissure
21	Corpus callosum, splenium
22	Fornix, crus
23	Choroidal fissure
24	Lateral ventricle, trigone (atrium)
25	Choroid plexus of lateral ventricle
26	Caudate nucleus, tail
27	Parietal operculum
28	Thalamus, laterodorsal nucleus (LD)
29	Thalamus, internal medullary lamina
30	Thalamostriate vein
31	Frontal operculum
32	Caudatolenticular gray bridges
33	Circular sulcus
34	Lateral ventricle, frontal (anterior) horn
35	Corpus callosum, forceps minor
36	Septum pellucidum, lamina
37	Anterior cerebral artery territory
38	Choroidal arteries territories
39	Middle cerbral artery territory
40	Posterior cerebral artery territory

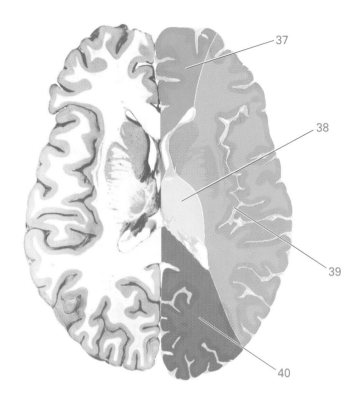

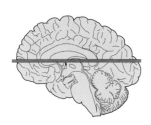

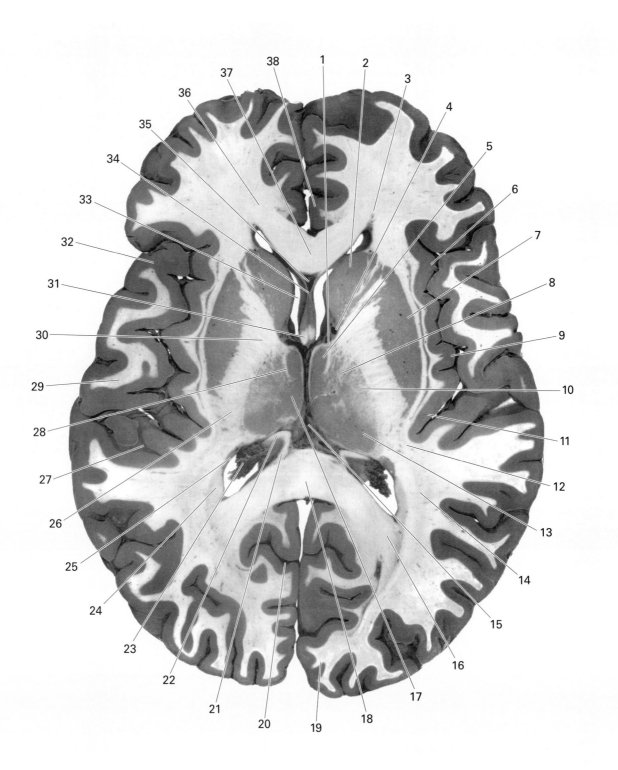

1	Thalamus, anterior thalamic peduncle
2	Caudate nucleus, head
3	Superior occipitofrontal fasciculus
4	Thalamostriate vein
5	Thalamus, anterior nucleus (A)
6	Insula, short gyrus
7	Putamen
8	Thalamus, ventroanterior nucleus (VA)
9	Insula, long gyrus
10	Thalamus, lateroposterior nucleus (LP)
11	Insula, long gyrus
12	Internal capsule, retrolenticular limb
13	Thalamus, pulvinar (Pul)
14	Optic radiation
15	Internal cerebral vein
16	Corpus callosum, forceps major
17	Thalamus, dorsomedial nucleus (DM)
18	Corpus callosum, splenium
19	Occipital lobe, cuneus
20	Calcarine fissure
21	Fornix, crus
22	Hippocampus, fimbria
23	Choroid plexus of lateral ventricle
24	Tapetum
25	Caudate nucleus, tail
26	Internal capsule, posterior limb
27	Circular sulcus
28	Thalamus, internal medullary lamina
29	Parietal operculum
30	Internal capsule, genu
31	Fornix, column
32	Frontal operculum
33	Lateral ventricle, frontal (anterior) horn
34	Septum pellucidum
35	Septum pellucidum, cavum
36	Corpus callosum, forceps minor
37	Corpus callosum, genu
38	Cingulate gyrus
39	Frontal operculum
40	Lateral ventricle, occipital (posterior) horn
41	Velum interpositum
42	Interventricular foramen (foramen of *Monro*)
43	Internal capsule, anterior limb

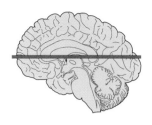

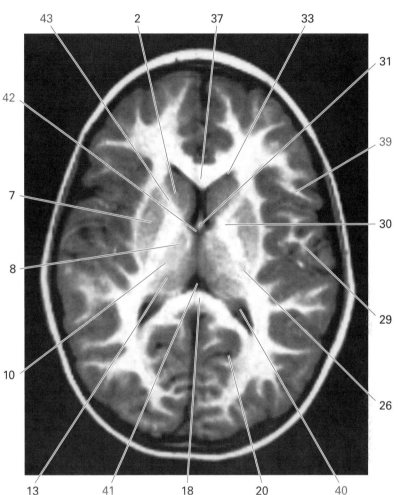

Brain Slices-Axial Sections

93

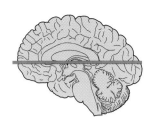

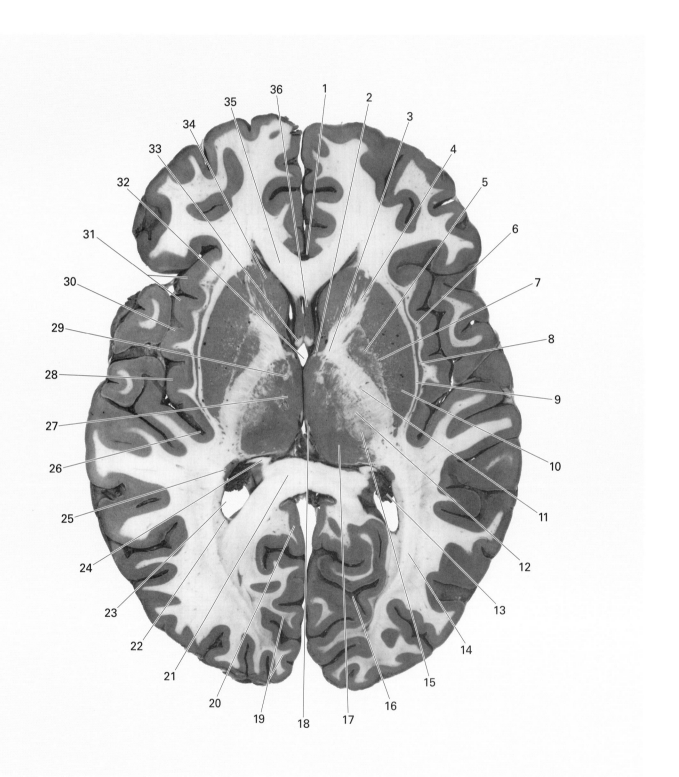

Axial Section Through Midlevel Diencephalon (1X) with Vessel Territories (0.7X)

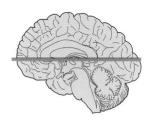

1	Anterior cerebral artery, pericallosal artery
2	Stria medullaris of thalamus
3	Internal capsule, genu
4	Internal capsule, anterior limb
5	Globus pallidus, external (lateral) segment (GPe)
6	Extreme capsule
7	Globus pallidus, lateral medullary lamina
8	Claustrum
9	External capsule
10	Putamen
11	Internal capsule, posterior limb
12	Thalamus, ventral posterolateral nucleus (VPL)
13	Choroid plexus of lateral ventricle
14	Optic radiation
15	Thalamus, centromedian nucleus (CM)
16	Calcarine fissure
17	Thalamus, pulvinar (Pul)
18	Stria medullaris of thalamus
19	Occipital lobe, cuneus
20	Cingulate gyrus
21	Corpus callosum, splenium
22	Tapetum
23	Lateral ventricle, trigone (atrium)
24	Hippocampus, fimbria
25	Caudate nucleus, tail
26	Circular sulcus
27	Thalamus, dorsomedial nucleus (DM)
28	Insula, long gyrus
29	Mamillothalamic tract
30	Precentral gyrus of insula
31	Insula, short gyri
32	Third ventricle (III)
33	Fornix, column
34	Caudate nucleus, head
35	Corpus callosum, genu
36	Septal nucleus
37	Anterior cerebral artery territory
38	Posterior communicating artery territory
39	Middle cerebral artery territory
40	Posterior cerebral artery, perforating branches territory
41	Choroidal arteries territory
42	Posterior cerebral artery territory

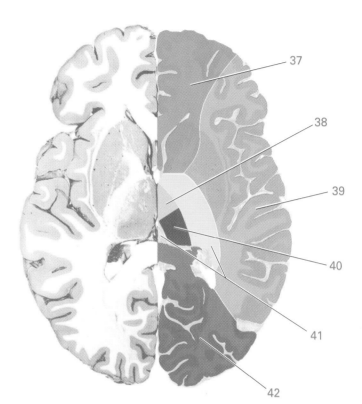

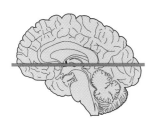

Axial Section Through Anterior Commissure (1X) with MRI (0.7X)

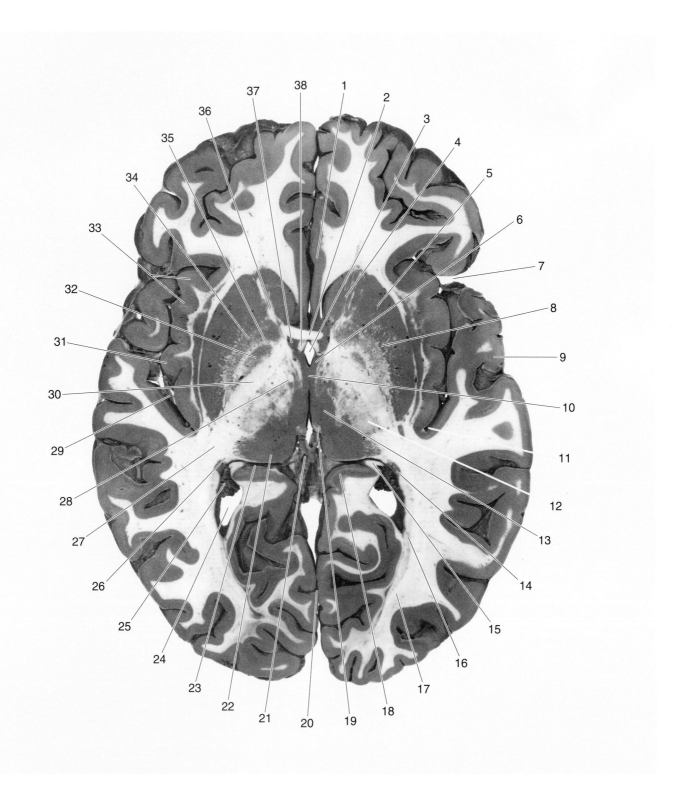

1	Cingulate gyrus
2	Anterior commissure
3	Third ventricle (III)
4	Caudate nucleus, head
5	Putamen
6	Hypothalamus, paraventricular nucleus
7	Lateral sulcus (*Sylvian* fissure)
8	Globus pallidus, lateral medullary lamina
9	Temporal operculum
10	Interthalamic adhesion (massa intermedia)
11	Circular sulcus
12	Thalamus, ventrolateral nucleus (VL)
13	Thalamus, dorsomedial nucleus (DM)
14	Caudate nucleus, tail
15	Hippocampus, fimbria
16	Tapetum
17	Optic radiation
18	Hippocampus, tail
19	Stria medullaris of thalamus
20	Longitudinal cerebral (interhemispheric) fissure
21	Great cerebral vein (vein of *Galen*)
22	Thalamus, pulvinar (Pul)
23	Choroidal fissure
24	Lateral ventricle, trigone (atrium)
25	Choroid plexus of lateral ventricle
26	Thalamo-occipital fasciculus
27	Internal capsule, retrolenticular part
28	Mamillothalamic tract
29	Middle cerebral artery, branch
30	Internal capsule, posterior limb
31	Insula, long gyrus
32	Globus pallidus, internal (medial) segment (GPi)
33	Insula, short gyri
34	Globus pallidus, external (lateral) segment (GPe)
35	Globus pallidus, medial medullary lamina
36	Internal capsule, anterior limb
37	Hypothalamus, lateral preoptic nucleus
38	Fornix, column
39	External capsule
40	Extreme capsule
41	Claustrum

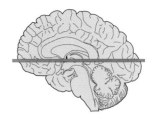

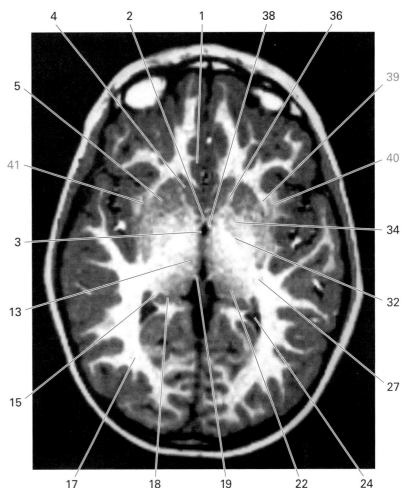

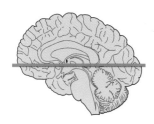

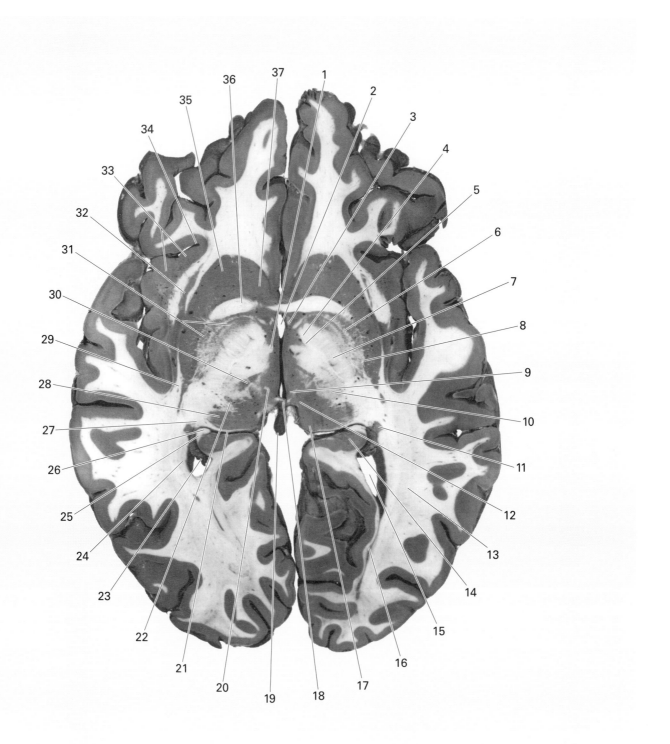

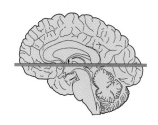

1	Mamillothalamic tract
2	Third ventricle (III)
3	Fornix, column
4	Lenticular fasciculus (H2 field of *Forel*)
5	Zona incerta
6	Globus pallidus, medial medullary lamina
7	Internal capsule, posterior limb
8	Globus pallidus, lateral medullary lamina
9	Habenula, medial nucleus
10	Thalamus, centromedian nucleus (CM)
11	Caudate nucleus, tail
12	Habenula, lateral nucleus
13	Inferior longitudinal fasciculus
14	Hippocampus
15	Lateral ventricle, occipital (posterior) horn
16	Corpus callosum, radiations
17	Thalamus, pulvinar (Pul)
18	Habenular commissure
19	Pineal gland
20	Habenulo-interpeduncular tract (fasciculus retroflexus of *Meynert*)
21	Thalamus, stratum zonale
22	Thalamus, ventroposterolateral nucleus (VPL)
23	Choroid plexus of lateral ventricle
24	Tapetum
25	Hippocampus, alveus
26	Hippocampus, fimbria
27	Stria terminalis
28	Thalamus, pulvinar (Pul)
29	External capsule
30	Thalamus, ventroposteromedial nucleus (VPM)
31	Globus pallidus, external (lateral) and internal (medial) segments (GPe and GPi)
32	Claustrum
33	Insula, short gyri
34	Circular suclus
35	Putamen
36	Anterior commissure
37	Caudate nucleus, head
38	Anterior cerebral artery territory
39	Posterior communicating artery territory
40	Posterior cerebral artery, perforating branches territory
41	Choroidal arteries territory
42	Middle cerebral artery territory
43	Posterior cerebral artery, collicular and posterior choroidal branches territory
44	Posterior cerebral artery territory

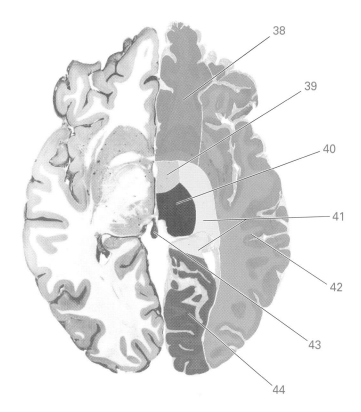

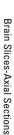

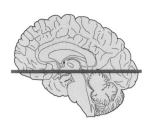

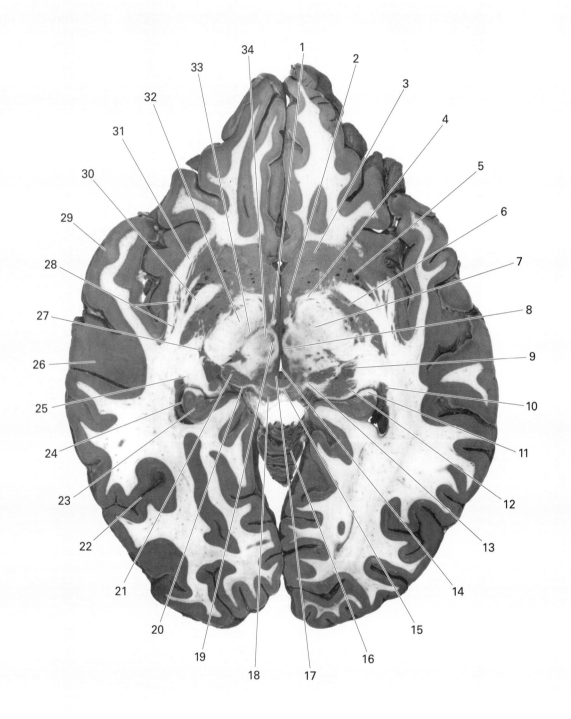

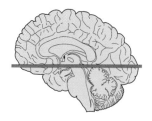

1	Mamillothalamic tract
2	Fornix, column
3	Caudate nucleus, head
4	Ansa lenticularis
5	Putamen
6	Globus pallidus external (lateral) segment (GPe)
7	Subthalamic nucleus
8	Capsule of red nucleus
9	Thalamus, dorsal lateral geniculate nucleus (dLGN) (lateral geniculate body)
10	Caudate nucleus, tail
11	Hippocampus, fimbria
12	Thalamus, pulvinar (Pul)
13	Superior colliculus, brachium
14	Cerebral aqueduct (aquaduct of *Sylvius*)
15	Commissure of superior colliculi
16	Cerebellum, vermis
17	Periaqueductal (central) gray substance
18	Superior colliculus
19	Habenulo-interpeduncular tract (fasciculus retroflexus of *Meynert*)
20	Capsule of medial geniculate nucleus (MG) (fibers from brachium of superior colliculus)
21	Thalamus, medial geniculate nucleus (MG) (medial geniculate body)
22	Middle temporal sulcus
23	Dentate gyrus
24	Hippocampus, alveus
25	Stria terminalis
26	Middle temporal gyrus
27	Thalamus, pregeniculate nucleus
28	Claustrum
29	Superior temporal gyrus
30	Anterior commissure
31	External capsule
32	Internal capsule, posterior limb
33	Zona incerta
34	Red nucleus
35	Gyrus rectus (straight gyrus)
36	Insula
37	Middle cerebral artery branch
38	Lateral ventricle, temporal (inferior) horn
39	Longitudinal cerebral (interhemispheric) fissure
40	Quadrigeminal cistern

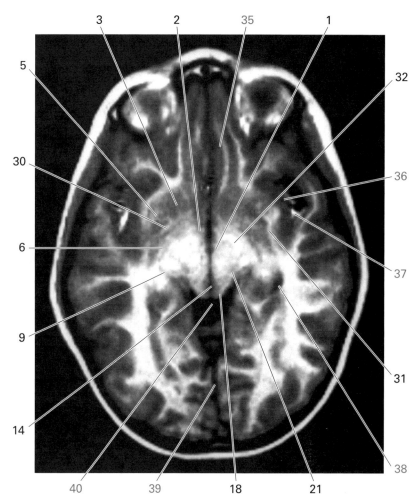

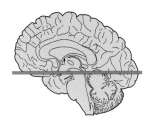

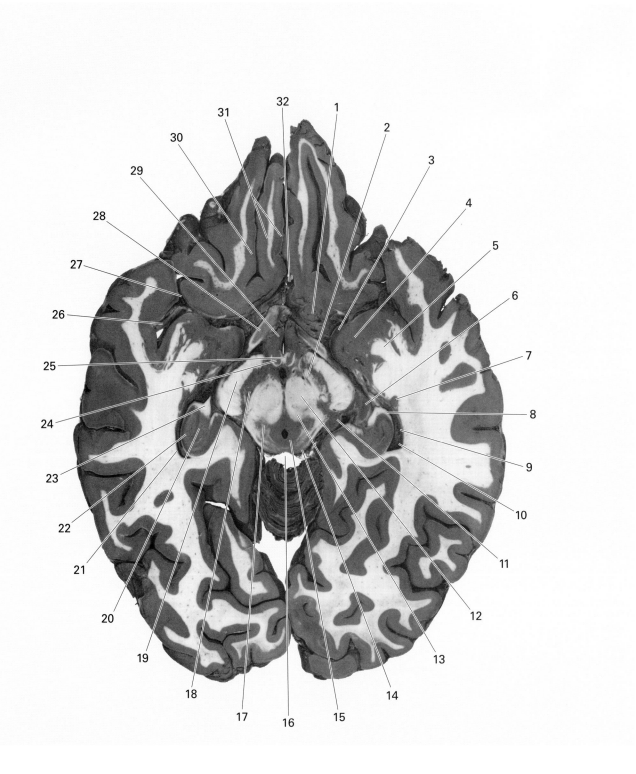

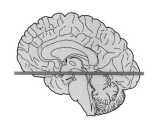

1 Anterior perforated substance
2 Mamillothalamic tract
3 Uncus
4 Amygdala
5 Anterior commissure
6 Thalamus, dorsal lateral geniculate nucleus (dLGN) (lateral geniculate body)
7 Caudate nucleus, tail
8 Hippocampus, alveus
9 Lateral ventricle, temporal (inferior) horn
10 Choroid plexus of lateral ventricle, temporal (inferior) horn
11 Thalamus, medial geniculate nucleus (MG) (medial geniculate body)
12 Red nucleus
13 Medial longitudinal fasciculus
14 Superior colliculus
15 Periaqueductal (central) gray substance
16 Ambient (circum-mesencephalic) cistern
17 Reticular formation (cuneiform nucleus)
18 Substantia nigra
19 Cerebral peduncle
20 Dentate gyrus
21 Tapetum
22 Hippocampus
23 Hippocampus, fimbria
24 Mamillary body
25 Principal mamillary fasciculus
26 Middle cerebral artery, branch
27 Lateral sulcus (*Sylvian* fissure)
28 Optic tract
29 Tuber cinereum
30 Medial orbital gyrus
31 Gyrus rectus (straight gyrus)
32 Anterial cerebral artery
33 Anterior cerebral artery territory
34 Internal carotid artery territory
35 Posterior communicating artery territory
36 Choroidal arteries territory
37 Middle cerebral artery territory
38 Posterior cerebral artery, perforating branches territory
39 Posterior cerebral artery, collicular and posterior choroidal branches territory
40 Posterior cerebral artery territory
41 Superior cerebellar artery territory

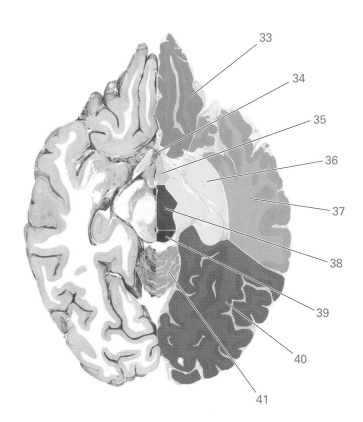

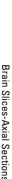

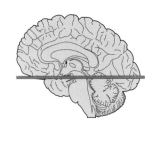

Axial Section Through Inferior Colliculi (1X) with MRI (0.7X)

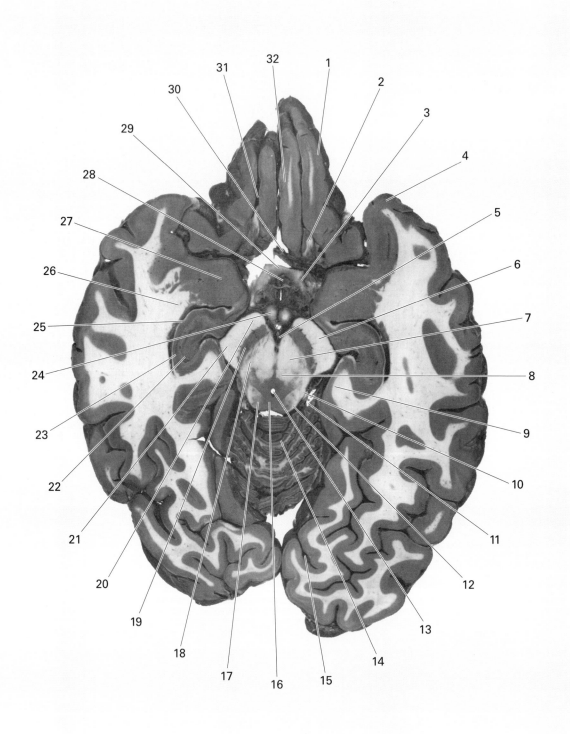

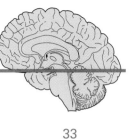

1	Medial orbital gyrus
2	Olfactory tract
3	Optic tract
4	Temporal pole
5	Interpeduncular fossa
6	Cerebral peduncle, corticospinal (pyramidal) tract
7	Superior cerebellar peduncle (brachium conjunctivum)
8	Medial longitudinal fasciculus
9	Parahippocampal gyrus
10	Lateral lemniscus
11	Ambient (circum-mesencephalic) cistern
12	Inferior colliculus, brachium
13	Cerebral aqueduct (aqueduct of *Sylvius*)
14	Cerebellum, vermis
15	Calcarine fissure
16	Periaqueductal (central) gray substance
17	Inferior colliculus
18	Medial lemniscus
19	Substantia nigra
20	Cerebral peduncle, (frontopontine tract)
21	Cerebral peduncle, (parietotemporo-occipitopontine tract)
22	Dentate gyrus
23	Hippocampus
24	Mamillary body
25	Hippocampus, alveus
26	Anterior commissure
27	Amygdala
28	Infundibulum (pituitary stalk)
29	Optic chiasm
30	Anterior cerebral artery
31	Olfactory sulcus
32	Gyrus rectus (straight gyrus)
33	Orbital fat
34	Superior sagittal sinus
35	Middle cerebral artery

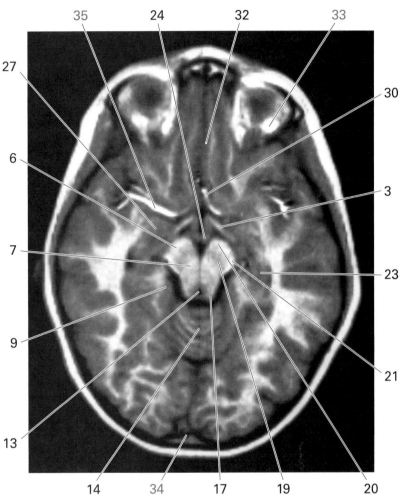

Brain Slices

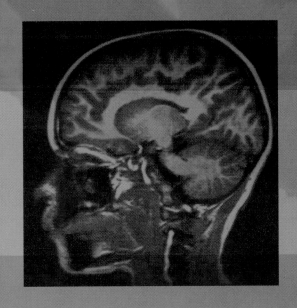

3. Sagittal Sections

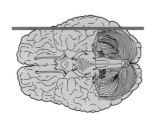

Sagittal Section Through Superior, Middle, and Inferior Temporal Gyri (1X) with Vessel Territories (0.7X)

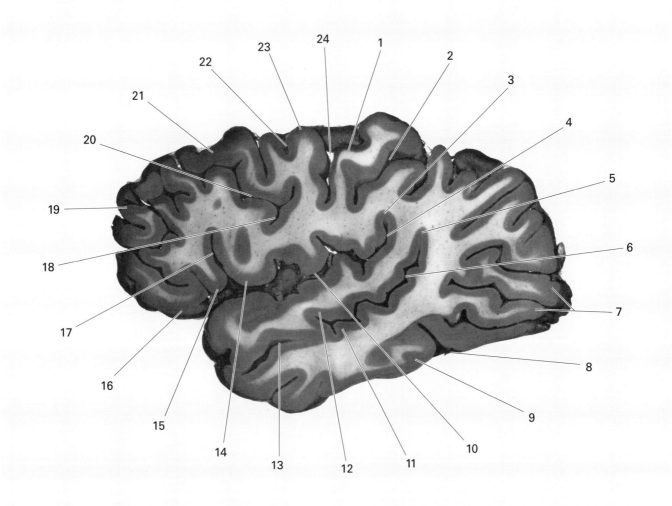

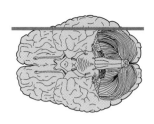

1	Postcentral gyrus
2	Postcentral sulcus
3	Supermarginal gyrus
4	Lateral sulcus (*Sylvian* fissure) posterior ascending limb (ramus)
5	Angular gyrus
6	Superior temporal sulcus
7	Occipital gyri
8	Preoccipital notch
9	Inferior temporal gyrus
10	Lateral sulcus (*Sylvian* fissure)
11	Middle temporal gyrus
12	Superior temporal gyrus
13	Superior temporal sulcus
14	Inferior frontal gyrus, opercular part
15	Inferior frontal gyrus, triangular part
16	Inferior fronal gyrus, orbital part
17	Lateral sulcus (*Sylvian* fissure), anterior ascending limb (ramus)
18	Precentral sulcus
19	Middle frontal gyrus
20	Superior frontal sulcus
21	Superior frontal gyrus
22	Precentral sulcus
23	Precentral gyrus
24	Central sulcus (fissure of *Rolando*)
25	Middle cerebral artery territory
26	Posterior cerebral artery territory

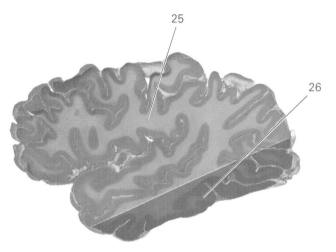

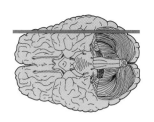
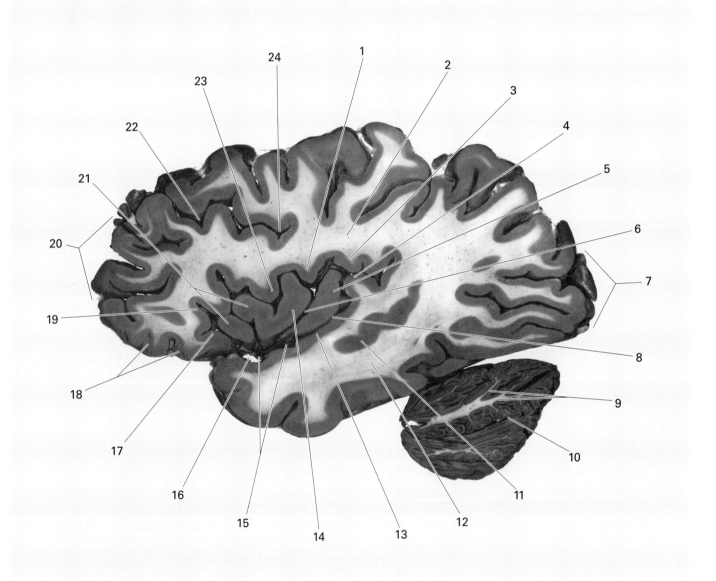

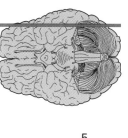

1	Precentral operculum
2	Centrum semiovale
3	Parietal operculum
4	Anterior transverse temporal gyrus
5	Insula, long gyrus
6	Insula, central fissure
7	Occipital lobe
8	Circular sulcus
9	Cerebellum, white matter
10	Cerebellum, horizontal fissure
11	Superior temporal sulcus
12	Optic radiation
13	Temporal operculum
14	Precentral gyrus of insula
15	Middle cerebral artery
16	Lateral sulcus (*Sylvian* fissure)
17	Orbital operculum
18	Orbital gyri
19	Inferior frontal gyrus
20	Frontal lobe
21	Insula, short gyri
22	Superior frontal sulcus
23	Frontal operculum
24	Precentral sulcus
25	Middle cerebral artery, branches
26	Orbital fat

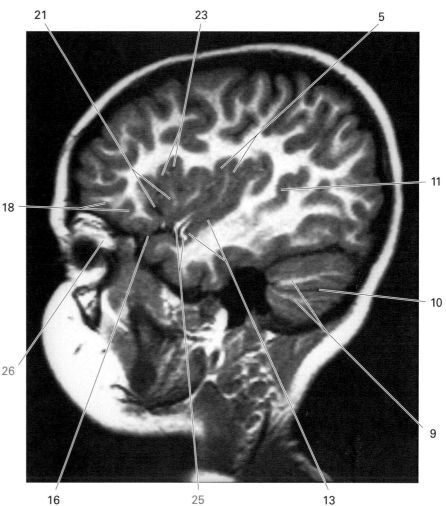

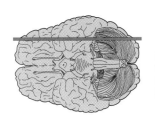

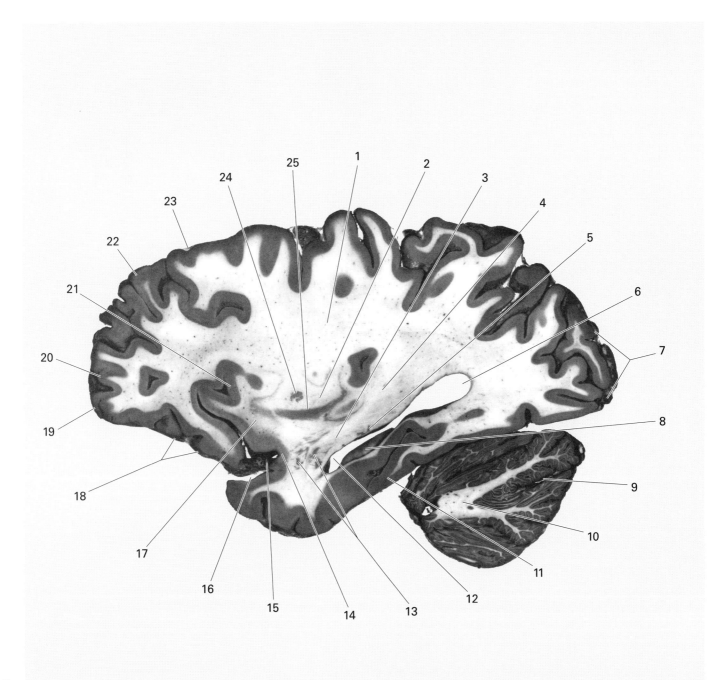

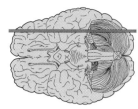

1 Centrum semiovale
2 External capsule
3 Optic radiation
4 Internal capsule, sublenticular limb (acoustic radiation)
5 Caudate nucleus, tail
6 Lateral ventricle, occipital (posterior) horn
7 Occipital lobe
8 Hippocampus
9 Cerebellum, horizontal fissure
10 Cerebellum, white matter
11 Lateral occipitotemporal gyrus
12 Lateral ventricle, temporal (inferior) horn
13 Amygdala
14 Limen of insula (stem of temporal lobe)
15 Middle cerebral artery
16 Lateral sulcus (*Sylvian* fissure)
17 Extreme capsule
18 Orbital gyri
19 Frontal pole
20 Inferior frontal gyrus
21 Insula
22 Middle frontal gyrus
23 Superior frontal gyrus
24 Putamen
25 Claustrum
26 Middle cerebral artery territory
27 Posterior cerebral artery territory
28 Superior cerebellar artery territory
29 Posterior inferior cerebellar artery territory
30 Anterior inferior cerebellar artery territory
31 Choroidal arteries territory
32 Anterior cerebral artery territory

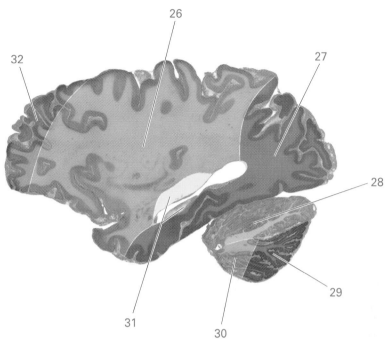

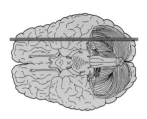

Sagittal Section Through Lateral Putamen (1X) with MRI (0.7X)

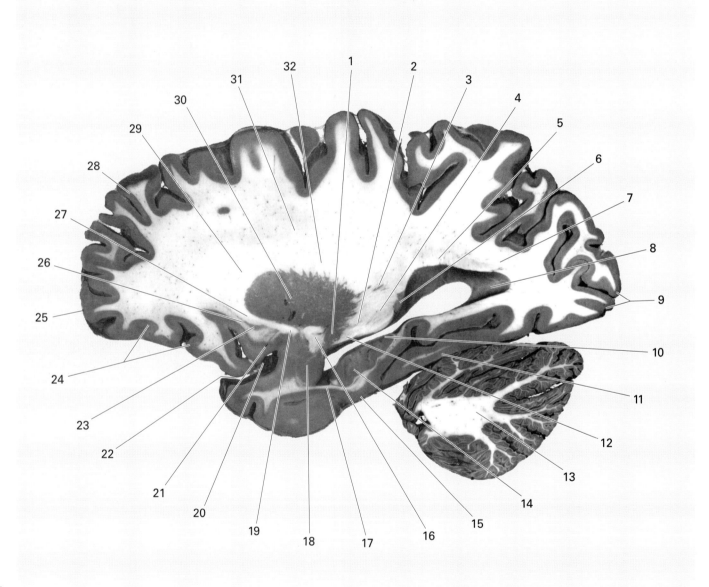

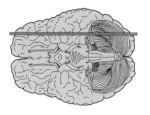

1 Putamen
2 Internal capsule, sublenticular limb (acoustic radiation)
3 Caudatolenticular gray bridges
4 Internal capsule, retrolenticular limb
5 Corpus callosum, forceps major
6 Caudate nucleus, tail
7 Optic radiation
8 Lateral ventricle, occipital (posterior) horn
9 Occipital gyri
10 Hippocampus, fimbria
11 Medial occipitotemporal (lingual) gyrus
12 Optic radiations
13 Cerebellum, white matter
14 Hippocampus
15 Parahippocampal gyrus
16 Anterior commissure
17 Cingulum
18 Amygdala
19 Uncinate fasciculus
20 Middle cerebral artery
21 Limen of insula (stem of temporal lobe)
22 Lateral sulcus (*Sylvian* fissure)
23 Claustrum
24 Orbital gyri
25 Frontal pole
26 Extreme capsule
27 External capsule
28 Middle frontal gyrus
29 Corona radiata
30 Putamen
31 Centrum semiovale
32 Corona radiata
33 Globus pallidus, external (lateral) segment (GPe)
34 Hippocampus, alveus
35 Internal carotid artery, intrapetrous part
36 Vertebral artery
37 Internal carotid artery, extracranial part
38 Maxillary air sinus
39 Inferior oblique and inferior rectus muscles
40 Levator palpebrae superioris muscle

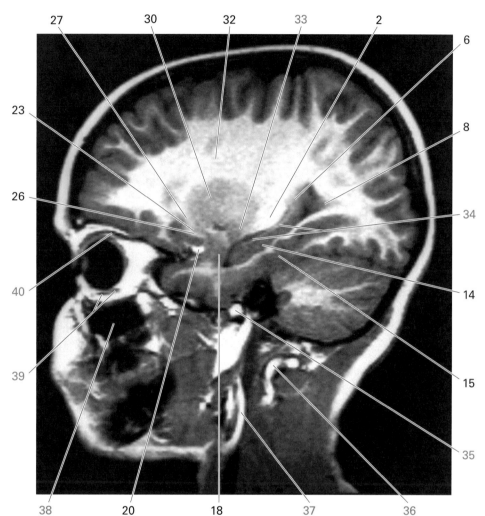

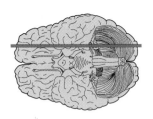

Sagittal Section Through Termination of Optic Tract (1X) with MRI (0.7X)

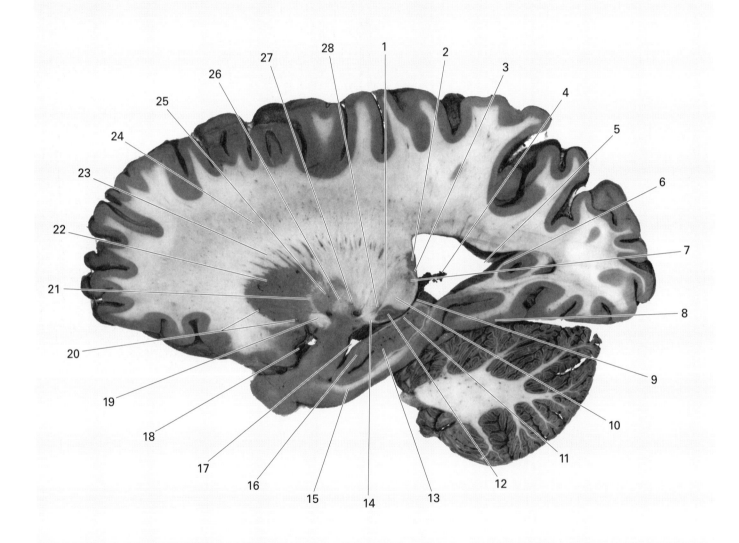

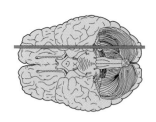

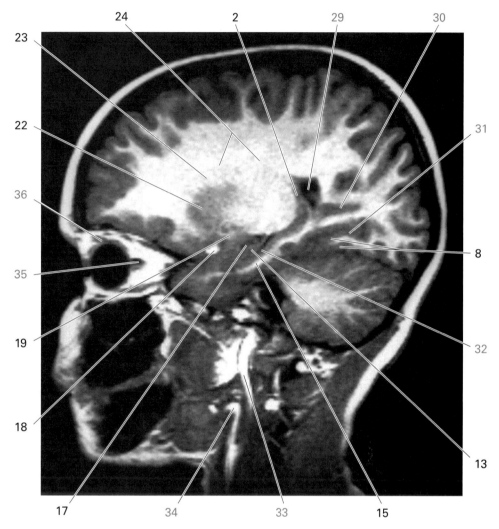

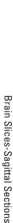

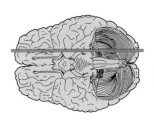

Sagittal Section Through Pulvinar (1X) with Vessel Territories (0.7X)

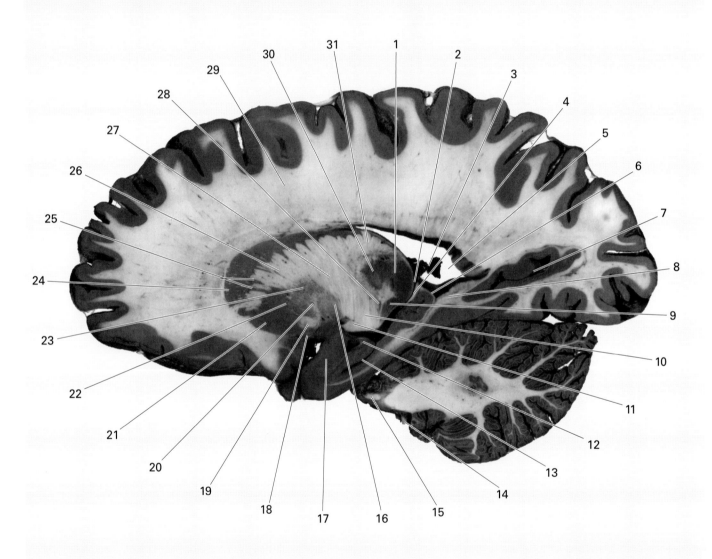

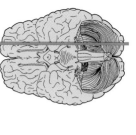

1   Thalamus, pulvinar (Pul)
2   Choroidal fissure
3   Choroid plexus
4   Hippocampus, fimbria
5   Lateral ventricle, trigone, (atrium)
6   Hippocampus, alveus
7   Calcarine fissure
8   Cingulum
9   Thalamus, dorsal lateral geniculate nucleus
    (dLGN) (lateral geniculate body)
10 Cerebral peduncle
11 Optic tract
12 Hippocampus, alveus
13 Hippocampal sulcus
14 Vestibulocochlear nerve (CN VIII)
15 Trigeminal nerve (CN V)
16 Globus pallidus, internal (medial) segment (GPi)
17 Amygdala
18 Lateral olfactory stria
19 Anterior commissure
20 Globus pallidus, medial medullary lamina
21 Putamen
22 Globus pallidus, lateral medullary lamina
23 Globus pallidus, external (lateral) segment (GPe)
24 Caudate nucleus, head
25 Caudatolenticular gray bridges
26 Internal capsule, anterior limb
27 Internal capsule, genu
28 Thalamus, reticular nucleus
29 Centrum semiovale
30 Thalamus, lateroposterior nucleus (LP)
31 Internal capsule, posterior limb
32 Middle cerebral artery territory
33 Posterior cerebral artery territory
34 Superior cerebellar artery territory
35 Posterior inferior cerebellar artery territory
36 Anterior inferior cerebellar artery territory
37 Posterior cerebral artery, perforating branches territory
38 Anterior cerebral artery territory
39 Choroidal arteries territory

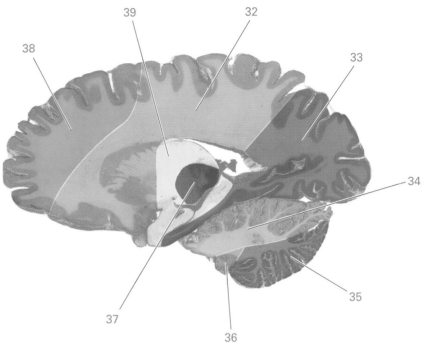

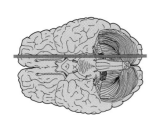

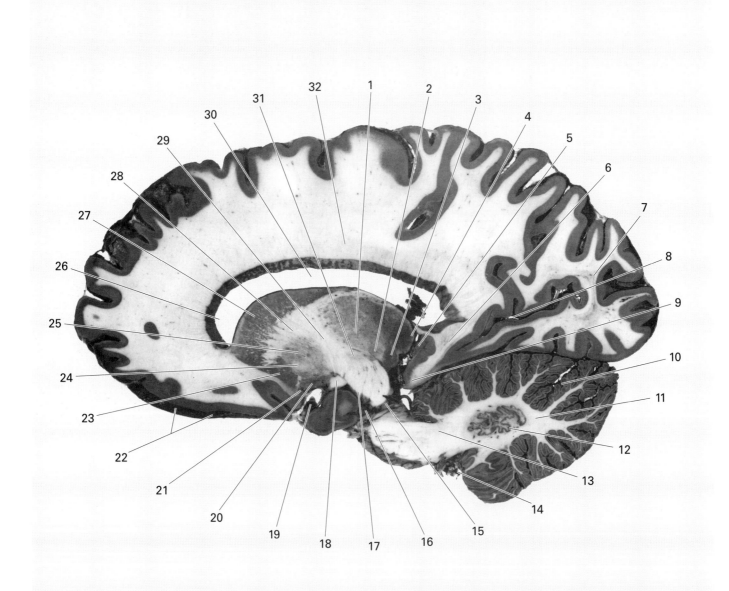

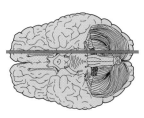

1	Thalamus, ventral lateral nucleus (VL)
2	Thalamus, ventral posterolateral nucleus (VPL)
3	Thalamus, medial geniculate nucleus (MG) (medial geniculate body)
4	Thalamus, pulvinar (Pul)
5	Hippocampus
6	Cingulum
7	Optic radiation
8	Calcarine sulcus
9	Parahippocampal gyrus
10	Semilunar lobule
11	Cerebellum, white matter
12	Dentate nucleus
13	Middle cerebellar peduncle (brachium pontis)
14	Fourth ventricle (IV), lateral aperture (foramen of *Luschka*)
15	Ambient (circum-mesencephalic) cistern
16	Posterior cerebral artery
17	Cerebral peduncle
18	Optic tract
19	Middle cerebral artery
20	Olfactory area
21	Olfactory tubercle
22	Orbital gyri
23	Putamen
24	Anterior commissure
25	Globus pallidus
26	Lateral ventricle, frontal (anterior) horn
27	Caudate nucleus, head
28	Internal capsule, anterior limb
29	Internal capsule, genu
30	Lateral ventricle, body
31	Subthalamic nucleus
32	Corpus callosum, body
33	Parieto-occipital sulcus
34	Cerebellum, horizontal fissure
35	Vertebral artery
36	Occipital condyle
37	Jugular tubercle
38	Carotid siphon
39	Medial rectus muscle

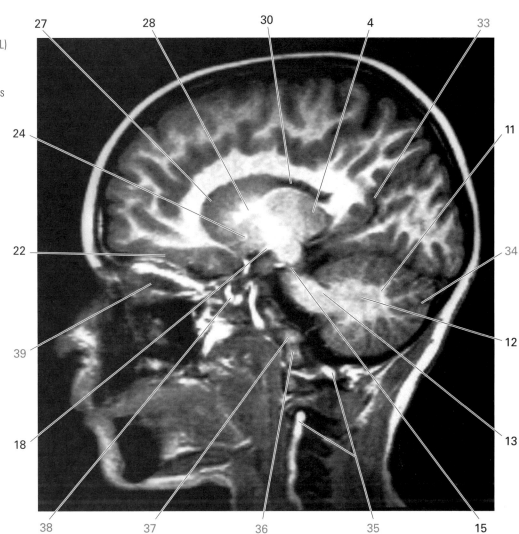

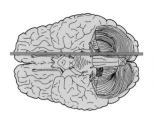

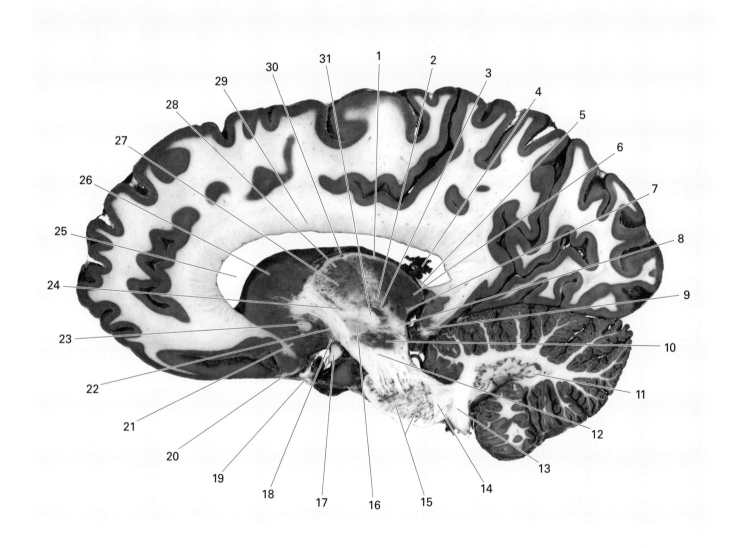

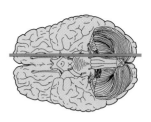

1   Thalamus, stratum zonale
2   Thalamus, centromedian nucleus (CM)
3   Thalamus, ventral posteromedial nucleus (VPM)
4   Choroid plexus
5   Fornix, crus
6   Thalamus, pulvinar (Pul)
7   Superior colliculus, brachium
8   Medial lemniscus
9   Posterior cerebral artery
10 Substantia nigra
11 Dentate nucleus
12 Cerebral peduncle
13 Inferior cerebellar peduncle (restiform body)
14 Middle cerebellar peduncle (brachium pontis)
15 Pontine nuclei (pontine gray)
16 Subthalamic nucleus
17 Optic tract
18 Ansa lenticularis
19 Internal carotid artery
20 Olfactory tract
21 Nucleus accumbens
22 Lenticular fasciculus (H$_2$ field of *Forel*)
23 Anterior commissure
24 Zona incerta
25 Lateral ventricle, frontal (anterior) horn
26 Caudate nucleus, head
27 Thalamus, ventral lateral nucleus (VL)
28 Thalamus, anterior nucleus (A)
29 Corpus callosum
30 Thalamostriate vein
31 Cerebellorubrothalamic tract
32 Posterior cerebral artery territory
33 Superior cerebellar artery territory
34 Posterior inferior cerebellar artery territory
35 Anterior inferior cerebellar artery territory
36 Basilar artery, lateral branches territory
37 Choroidal arteries territory
38 Anterior cerebral artery territory
39 Posterior cerebral artery, perforating branches territory

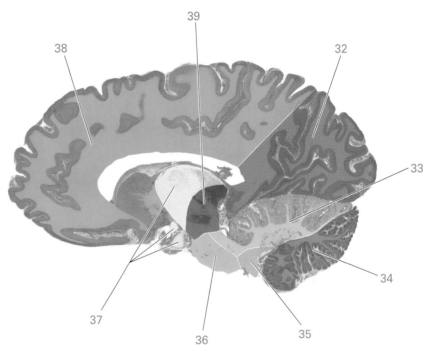

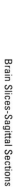

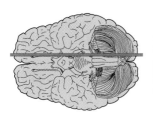

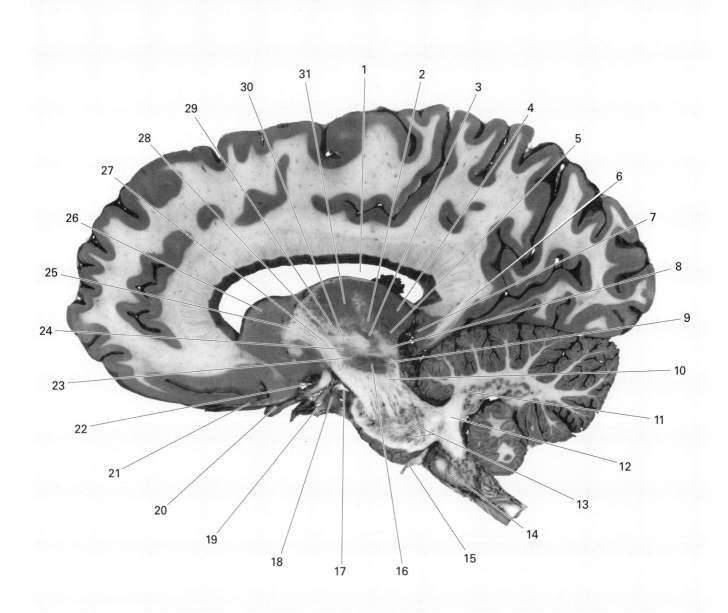

Sagittal Section Through Inferior Cerebellar Peduncle (Restiform Body) (1X) with Vessel Territories (0.7X)

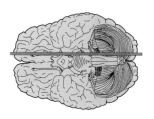

1	Lateral ventricle
2	Thalamus, centromedian nucleus (CM)
3	Thalamus, ventral posteromedial nucleus (VPM)
4	Thalamus, pulvinar (Pul)
5	Thalamus, medial geniculate nucleus (MG) (medial geniculate body)
6	Cingulum
7	Parahippocampal gyrus
8	Medial lemniscus
9	Pallidoreticular (lenticulonigral) tracts
10	Lateral corticobulbar fibers
11	Dentate nucleus
12	Inferior cerebellar peduncle (restiform body)
13	Pontine nuclei (pontine gray)
14	Inferior olive
15	Abducens nerve (CN VI)
16	Substantia nigra
17	Posterior cerebral artery
18	Uncus
19	Oculomotor nerve (CN III)
20	Optic nerve (CN II)
21	Olfactory tract
22	Anterior cerebral artery
23	Capsule of subthalamic nucleus
24	Subthalamic nucleus
25	Internal capsule, anterior limb
26	Caudate nucleus, head
27	Internal capsule, genu
28	Zona incerta
29	Thalamic fasciculus (H$_1$ field of *Forel*)
30	Lenticular fasciculus (H$_2$ field of *Forel*)
31	Thalamus, lateroposterior nucleus (LP)
32	Posterior cerebral artery, perforating branches territory
33	Posterior cerebral artery territory
34	Superior cerebellar artery territory
35	Posterior inferior cerebellar artery territory
36	Vertebral artery territory
37	Basilar artery, medial branches territory
38	Choroidal arteries territory
39	Internal carotid artery territory
40	Anterior cerebral artery territory
41	Posterior communicating artery territory

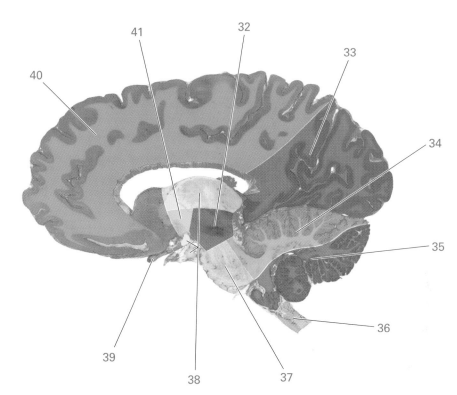

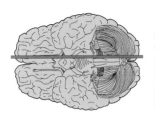

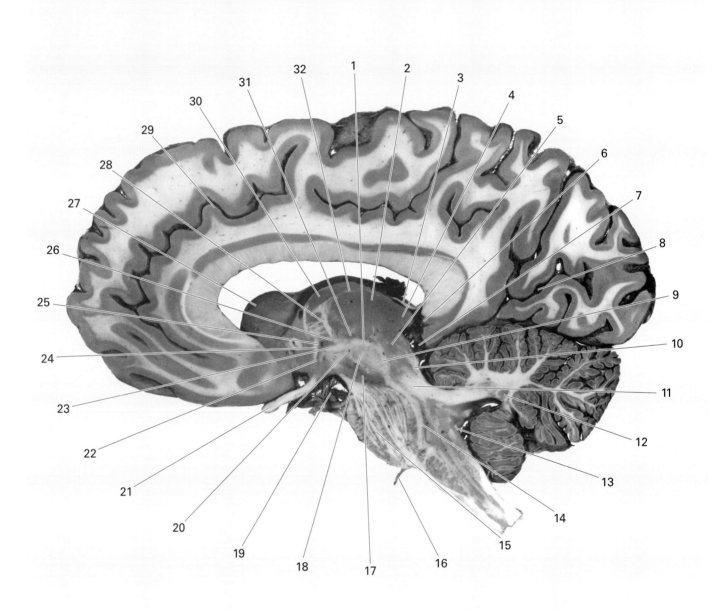

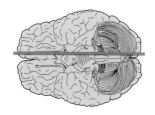

1 Thalamic fasciculus
   (H$_1$ field of *Forel*)
2 Thalamus, dorsomedial
   nucleus (DM)
3 Fornix, crus
4 Thalamus, pulvinar (Pul)
5 Pretectal area
6 Fasciolar gyrus
7 Posterior cerebral artery
8 Calcarine fissure
9 Medial lemniscus
10 Lateral lemniscus
11 Superior cerebellar peduncle
   (brachium conjuctivum)
12 Fastigial nucleus
13 Medullary striae of fourth
   ventricle (IV)
14 Medial lemniscus
15 Corticospinal (pyramidal) tract
16 Abducent nerve (CN VI)
17 Substantia nigra
18 Red nucleus
19 Posterior cerebral artery
20 Tegmental area H
   (H field of *Forel*)
21 Optic nerve (CN II)
22 Ansa lenticularis
23 Lenticular fasciculus
   (H$_2$ field of *Forel*)
24 Inferior thalamic peduncle
   (radiations)
25 Zona incerta
26 Thalamic fasciculus
   (H$_1$ field of *Forel*)
27 Caudate nucleus, head
28 Mamillothalamic tract
29 Cingulate sulcus
30 Thalamus, anterior nucleus (A)
31 Thalamus, ventral posteromedial nucleus (VPM)
32 Thalamus, internal medullary lamina
33 Fornix
34 Parieto-occipital sulcus
35 Calcarine fissure
36 Quadrigeminal cistern
37 Superior and inferior colliculi (quadrigeminal
   plate, tectum)

38 Cerebellum, tonsil
39 Vertebral artery
40 Pontine cistern
41 Clivus
42 Anterior cerebral artery
43 Gyrus rectus (straight gyrus)
44 Optic tract
45 Corpus callosum, body

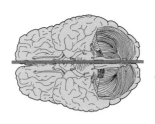

Sagittal Section Through Red Nucleus (1X) with Vessel Territories (0.7X)

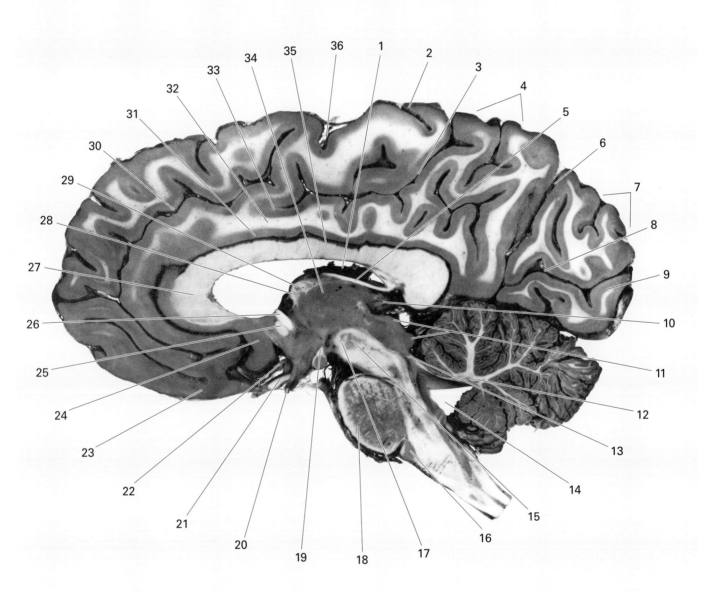

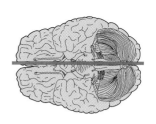

1 Choroid plexus of lateral ventricle
2 Central sulcus (fissure of *Rolando*)
3 Cingulate sulcus, marginal branch
4 Parietal lobe, precuneus
5 Fornix, body
6 Parieto-occipital sulcus
7 Occipital lobe, cuneus
8 Calcarine fissure
9 Medial occipitotemporal (lingual) gyrus
10 Pineal gland
11 Superior and inferior colliculi
   (quadrigeminal plate, tectum)
12 Fastigial nucleus
13 Trochlear nerve (CN IV), decussation
14 Fourth ventricle (IV)
15 Red nucleus
16 Arcuate nucleus
17 Habenulo-interpeduncular tract
   (fasciculus retroflexus of *Meynert*)
18 Pons
19 Principal mamillary fasciculus
20 Infundibulum (pituitary stalk)
21 Optic chiasm
22 Anterior cerebral artery
23 Gyrus rectus (straight gyrus)
24 Subcallosal area (gyrus)
25 Anterior commissure
26 Fornix, column
27 Corpus callosum, genu
28 Stria medullaris of thalamus
29 Thalamus, anterior nucleus (A)
30 Cingulate sulcus
31 Callosal sulcus
32 Cingulum
33 Cingulate gyrus
34 Thalamus, dorsomedial nucleus (DM)
35 Corpus callosum, body
36 Precentral sulcus
37 Posterior cerebral artery, collicular and posterior
   choroidal branches territory
38 Posterior cerebral artery territory
39 Superior cerebellar artery territory
40 Posterior inferior cerebellar artery territory
41 Posterior spinal artery territory
42 Anterior spinal artery territory
43 Basilar artery, medial branches territory

44 Posterior cerebral artery, perforating branches territory
45 Internal carotid artery territory
46 Posterior communicating artery territory
47 Anterior cerebral artery territory
48 Choroidal arteries territory

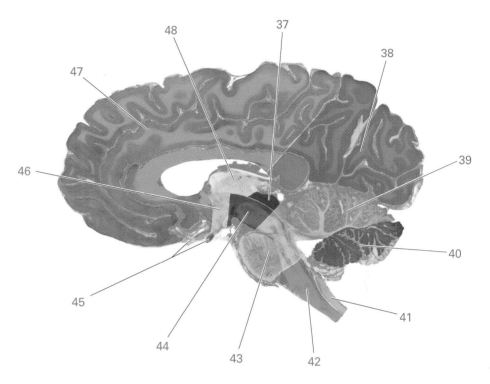

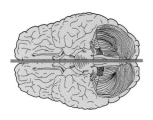

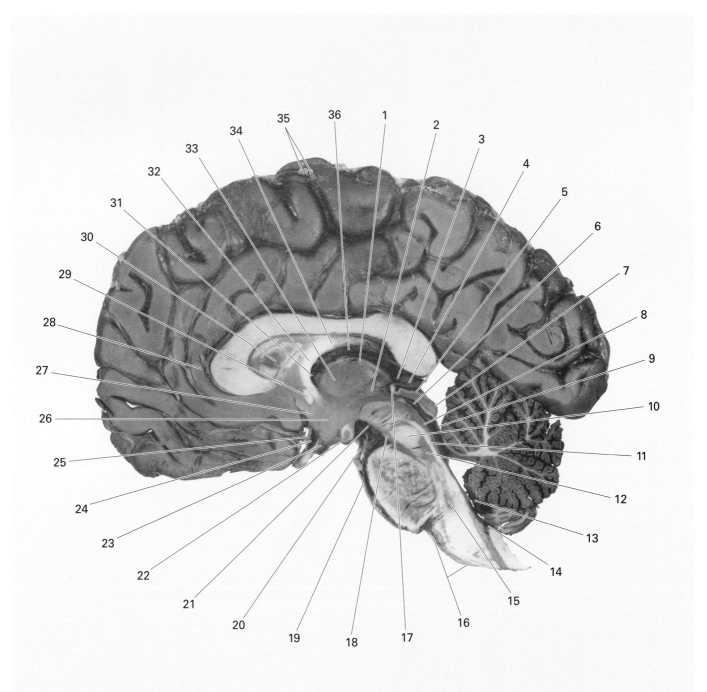

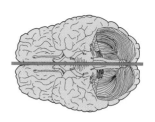

1	Stria medullaris of thalamus
2	Third ventricle (III)
3	Habenular commissure
4	Pineal gland
5	Superior colliculus
6	Cerebral aqueduct (aqueduct of *Sylvius*)
7	Inferior colliculus
8	Periaqueductal (central) gray substance
9	Superior medullary velum
10	Superior cerebellar peduncle (brachium conjunctivum), decussation
11	Medial longitudinal fasciculus
12	Superior central nucleus
13	Choroid plexus of fourth ventricle (IV)
14	Obex
15	Inferior central nucleus
16	Medulla oblongata
17	Posterior commissure
18	Interpeduncular nucleus
19	Basilar artery
20	Posterior cerebral artery, perforating branches
21	Posterior perforated substance
22	Mamillary body
23	Third ventricle (III), infundibular recess
24	Third ventricle (III), optic (supraoptic) recess
25	Lamina terminalis
26	Hypothalamus
27	Hypohalamus, preoptic area
28	Anterior cerebral artery, pericallosal artery
29	Anterior commissure
30	Septum pellucidum
31	Interventricular foramen (foramen of *Monro*)
32	Fornix, column
33	Thalamus, paraventricular nucleus
34	Fornix, body
35	Arachnoid granulations
36	Velum interpositum
37	Corpus callosum, splenium
38	Fourth ventricle (IV)
39	Cisterna magna
40	Pons
41	Clivus
42	Interpeduncular cistern
43	Optic chiasm
44	Corpus callosum, genu
45	Mamillothalamic tract

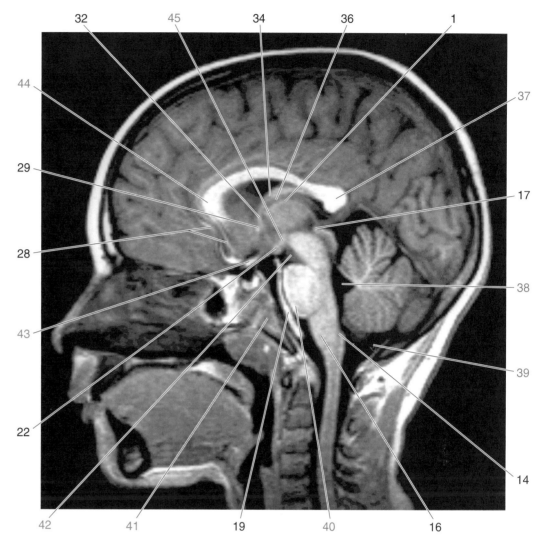

Histological Sections

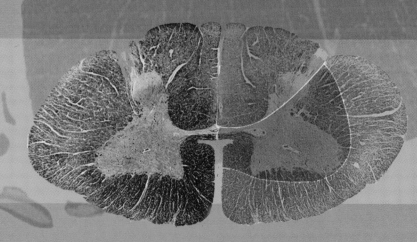

1. Spinal Cord

Transverse Section Through Sacral Spinal Cord (10X)

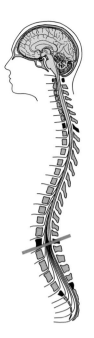

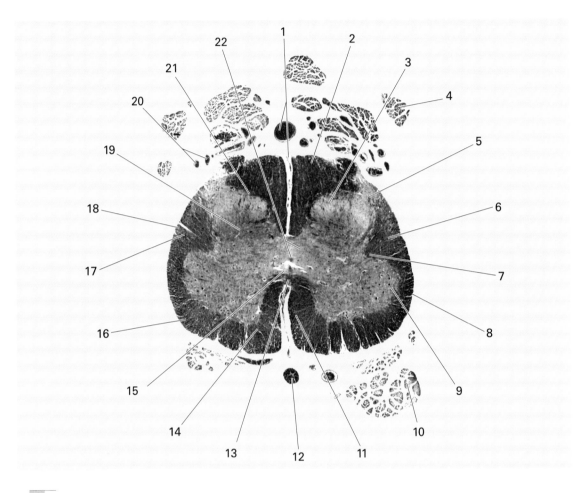

1	Dorsal (posterior) median sulcus and vein
2	Gracile fasciculus
3	Substantia gelatinosa (posterior [dorsal] horn)
4	Posterior (dorsal) root fibers (cauda equina)
5	Dorsolateral fasciculus (*Lissauer's* tract)
6	Lateral corticospinal tract
7	Lateral fasciculus proprius
8	Spinal lemniscus (spinoreticular, spinotectal, and spinothalamic tracts)
9	Anterior (ventral) horn, lateral motor nuclei
10	Anterior (ventral) root fibers (cauda equina)
11	Medial (pontine) reticulospinal tract
12	Anterior spinal artery
13	Anterior white commissure
14	Anterior fasciculus proprius
15	Anterior gray commissure
16	Lateral spinothalamic tract
17	Lateral (medullary) reticulospinal tract
18	Posterior (dorsal) spinocerebellar tract
19	Nucleus proprius
20	Posterior (dorsal) spinal artery and branch
21	Marginal nucleus
22	Central canal and dorsal gray commissure

Transverse Section Through Lumbar Enlargement of Spinal Cord (10X) with Vessel Territories

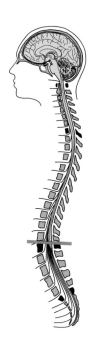

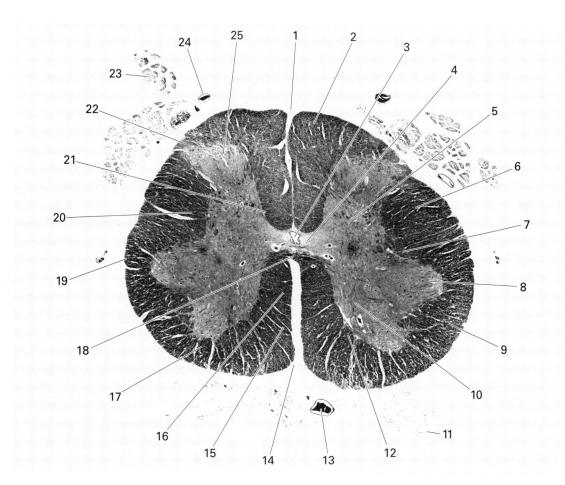

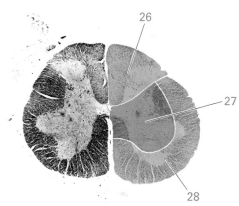

1	Posterior (dorsal) median sulcus	21	Posterior (dorsal) fasciculus proprius
2	Gracile fasciculus	22	Dorsolateral fasciculus (*Lissauer's* tract)
3	Central canal	23	Posterior (dorsal) root fibers
4	Posterior gray commissure	24	Posterior (dorsal) spinal artery
5	Nucleus proprius	25	Substantia gelatinosa (posterior [dorsal] horn)
6	Lateral corticospinal tract	26	Posterior spinal artery territory
7	Lateral fasciculus proprius	27	Anterior spinal artery territory
8	Anterior (ventral) horn, lateral motor nuclei	28	Radicular arteries territory
9	Spinal lemniscus (spinoreticular, spinotectal, and spinothalamic tracts)		
10	Anterior (ventral) horn, medial motor nuclei		
11	Anterior (ventral) root fibers (cauda equina)		
12	Anterior fasciculus proprius		
13	Anterior spinal artery		
14	Anterior (ventral) median fissure (sulcus)		
15	Medial (pontine) reticulospinal tract		
16	Anterior corticospinal tract		
17	Lateral vestibulospinal tract		
18	Anterior white commissure		
19	Anterior (ventral) spinocerebellar tract		
20	Rubrospinal tract		

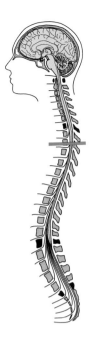

Transverse Section Through Thoracic Spinal Cord (10X) with Vessel Territories

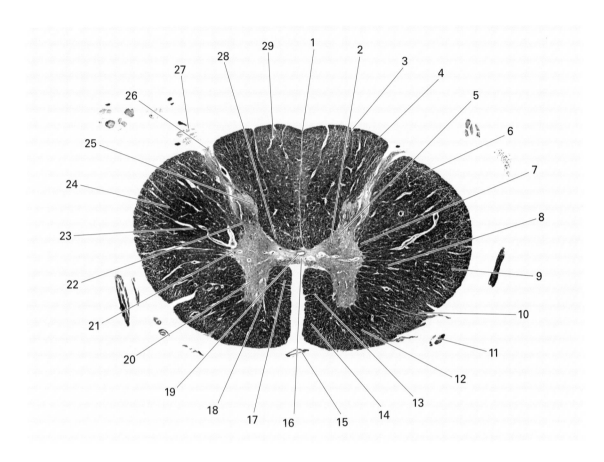

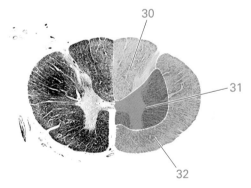

1	Raphé
2	Dorsal (posterior) nucleus (*Clarke's* column)
3	Posterior (dorsal) intermediate sulcus (paramedian sulcus)
4	Cuneate fasciculus
5	Nucleus proprius
6	Posterior (dorsal) spinocerebellar tract
7	Lateral fasciculus proprius
8	Lateral (medullary) reticulospinal tract
9	Anterior (ventral) spinocerebellar tract
10	Spinal lemniscus (spinoreticular, spinotectal, and spinothalamic tracts)
11	Anterior (ventral) root
12	Spinothalamic tracts
13	Medial (pontine) reticulospinal tract
14	Anterior corticospinal tract
15	Anterior spinal artery
16	Anterior gray commissure
17	Medial longitudinal fasciculus
18	Anterior (ventral) rootlets
19	Central canal
20	Anterior (ventral) horn, medial motor nuclei
21	Lateral horn, intermediolateral cell column (nucleus)
22	Posterior (dorsal) horn

23	Rubrospinal tract
24	Lateral corticospinal tract
25	Substantia gelatinosa (posterior [dorsal] horn)
26	Dorsolateral fasciculus (*Lissauer's* tract)
27	Posterior (dorsal) root fibers
28	Posterior (dorsal) fasciculus proprius
29	Gracile fasciculus
30	Posterior spinal artery territory
31	Anterior spinal artery territory
32	Radicular arteries territory

Transverse Section Through Cervical Enlargement of Spinal Cord (10X) with Vessel Territories

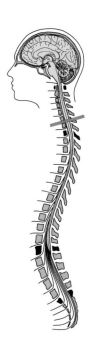

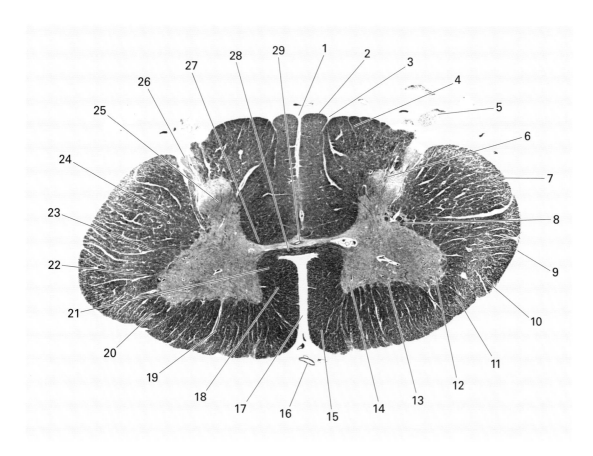

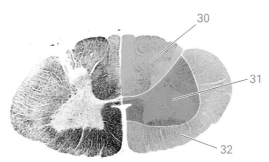

1	Posterior (dorsal) median sulcus	
2	Gracile fasciculus	
3	Posterior (dorsal) intermediate sulcus (paramedian sulcus)	
4	Cuneate fasciculus	
5	Posterior (dorsal) root fibers	
6	Substantia gelatinosa (posterior [dorsal] horn)	
7	Posterior (dorsal) spinocerebellar tract	
8	Lateral fasciculus proprius	
9	Anterior (ventral) spinocerebellar tract	
10	Spino-olivary tract	
11	Spinal lemniscus (spinoreticular, spinotectal, and spinothalamic tracts)	
12	Anterior (ventral) horn, lateral motor nuclei	
13	Anterior (ventral) fasciculus proprius	
14	Anterior (ventral) horn, medial motor nuclei	
15	Anterior corticospinal tract	
16	Anterior spinal artery	
17	Anterior (ventral) median fissure (sulcus)	
18	Tectospinal tract	
19	Medial (pontine) reticulospinal tract	
20	Lateral vestibulospinal tract	
21	Medial vestibulospinal tract (medial longitudinal fasciculus)	

22	Lateral (medullary) reticulospinal tract
23	Rubrospinal tract
24	Lateral corticospinal tract
25	Nucleus proprius
26	Dorsolateral fasciculus (*Lissauer's* tract)
27	Posterior (dorsal) fasciculus proprius
28	Anterior (ventral) white commissure
29	Central canal
30	Posterior spinal artery territory
31	Anterior spinal artery territory
32	Radicular arteries territory

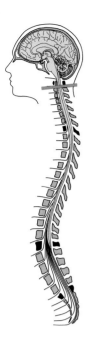

Transverse Section Through Upper Cervical Spinal Cord (10X)

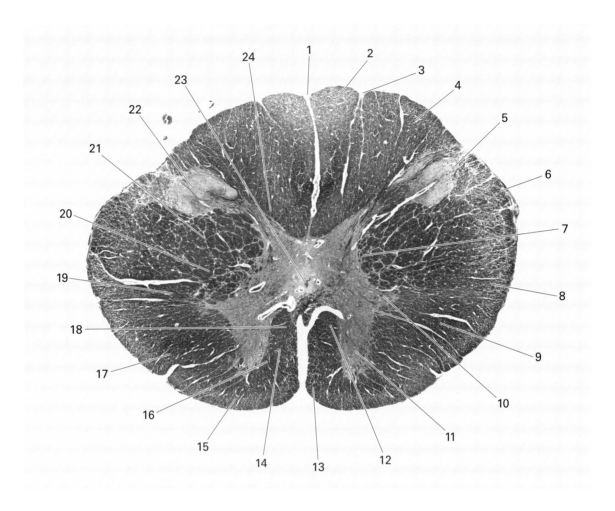

1	Posterior (dorsal) median sulcus	13	Anterior corticospinal tract
2	Gracile fasciculus	14	Tectospinal tract
3	Posterior (dorsal) intermediate sulcus (paramedian sulcus)	15	Medial (pontine) reticulospinal tract
		16	Anterior fasciculus proprius
4	Cuneate fasciculus	17	Lateral vestibulospinal tract
5	Marginal nucleus	18	Medial vestibulospinal tract (medial longitudinal fasciculus)
6	Posterior (dorsal) spinocerebellar tract		
7	Lateral fasciculus proprius	19	Lateral (medullary) reticulospinal tract
8	Anterior (ventral) spinocerebellar tract	20	Rubrospinal tract
9	Spinal lemniscus (spinoreticular, spinotectal, and spinothalamic tracts)	21	Lateral corticospinal tract
		22	Substantia gelatinosa (posterior [dorsal] horn)
10	Accessory nucleus (CN XI)	23	Central canal
11	Anterior (ventral) horn, medial motor nuclei	24	Posterior (dorsal) fasciculus proprius
12	Medial longitudinal fasciculus		

Part IV

Histological Sections

2. Brain Stem and Cerebellum

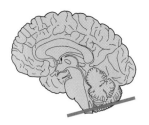

Transverse Section Through Decussation of Pyramids (5X)

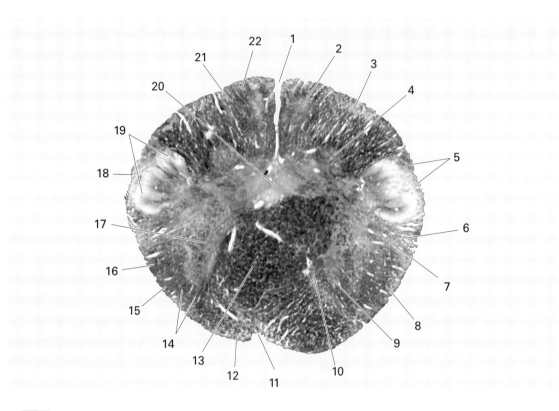

1	Posterior (dorsal) median sulcus
2	Gracile nucleus
3	Cuneate fasciculus
4	Cuneate nucleus
5	Trigeminal nerve (CN V), spinal tract
6	Posterior (dorsal) spinocerebellar tract
7	Rubrospinal tract
8	Anterior (ventral) spinocerebellar tract
9	Anterior (ventral) horn, medial motor nuclei
10	Medial longitudinal fasciculus
11	Anterior (ventral) median fissure (sulcus)
12	Pyramids (corticospinal tracts)
13	Pyramidal decussation (corticospinal tracts)
14	Medial (pontine), lateral (medullary) reticulospinal tracts and lateral vestibulospinal tract
15	Spino-olivary tract
16	Spinal lemniscus (spinothalamic, spinotectal, and spinoreticular tracts)
17	Spinal accessory nucleus (CN XI)
18	Trigeminal eminence
19	Trigeminal (CN V) spinal nucleus
20	Central gray
21	Posterior (dorsal) intermediate sulcus (paramedian sulcus)
22	Gracile fasciculus

Transverse Section Through Inferior Olive (5X) with Vessel Territories

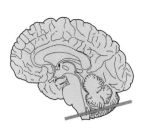

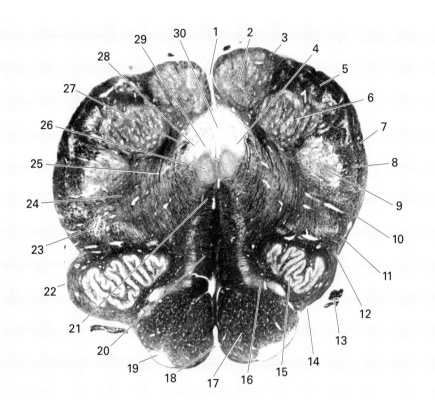

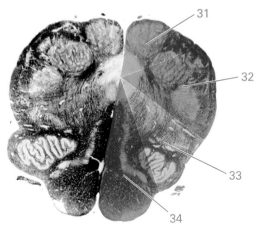

1	Posterior (dorsal) median sulcus
2	Gracile nucleus
3	Gracile fasciculus
4	Dorsal (posterior) motor nucleus of vagus (CN X)
5	Cuneate fasciculus
6	Cuneate nucleus
7	Posterior (dorsal) spinocerebellar tract
8	Trigeminal nerve (CN V), spinal tract
9	Trigeminal (CN V) spinal nucleus
10	Anterior (ventral) spinocerebellar tract
11	Rubrospinal tract
12	Spinal lemniscus (spinoreticular, spinotectal, and spinothalamic tracts)
13	Accessory nerve (CN XI), spinal root
14	External arcuate fibers
15	Inferior olivary nucleus
16	Medial accessory olivary nucleus
17	Corticospinal (pyramidal) tract
18	Anterior (ventral) median fissure (sulcus)
19	Arcuate nucleus
20	Medial lemniscus
21	Medial longitudinal fasciculus
22	Olivary eminence
23	Lateral reticular nucleus
24	Nucleus ambiguus (ventral motor nucleus of vagus) (CN X)

25	Internal arcuate fibers and bulbar reticular formation
26	Hypoglossal nucleus (CN XII)
27	Solitary tract
28	Solitary nucleus
29	Posterior (dorsal) longitudinal fasciculus
30	Central canal
31	Posterior spinal artery territory
32	Posterior inferior cerebellar artery territory
33	Vertebral artery territory
34	Anterior spinal artery territory

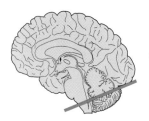

Transverse Section Through Hypoglossal Nucleus (5X) with Vessel Territories

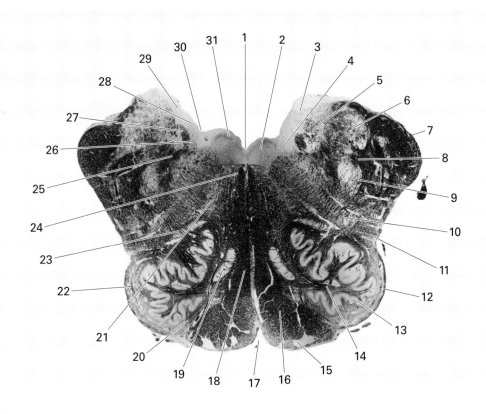

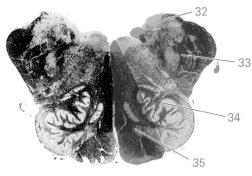

1	Median sulcus of fourth ventricle (IV)
2	Hypoglossal nucleus (CN XII)
3	Medial vestibular nucleus (CN VIII)
4	Dorsal (posterior) motor nucleus of vagus (CN X)
5	Inferior vestibular nucleus (CN VIII)
6	Accessory (lateral) cuneate nucleus
7	Inferior cerebellar peduncle, (restiform body)
8	Trigeminal nerve (CN V), spinal tract
9	Trigeminal (CN V) spinal nucleus
10	Nucleus ambiguus (ventral motor nucleus of vagus) (CN X)
11	Spinal lemniscus (spinoreticular, spinotectal, and spinothalamic tracts)
12	Olivary eminence
13	Inferior olivary nucleus
14	Inferior olive (hilum)
15	Arcuate nucleus
16	Corticospinal (pyramidal) tract
17	Anterior (ventral) median fissure (sulcus)
18	Medial lemniscus
19	Medial accessory olivary nucleus
20	Hypoglossal nerve root (CN XII)
21	Medullary reticular formation (gigantocellular nucleus) and central tegmental tract
22	External arcuate fibers

23	Dorsal accessory olivary nucleus
24	Medial longitudinal fasciculus
25	Vagus nerve (CN X), root
26	Solitary nucleus
27	Solitary tract
28	Area postrema
29	Periventricular gray substance
30	Limiting sulcus of fourth ventricle (IV) (sulcus limitans)
31	Dorsal longitudinal fasciculus
32	Anterior inferior cerebellar artery territory
33	Posterior inferior cerebellar artery territory
34	Vertebral artery territory
35	Anterior spinal artery territory

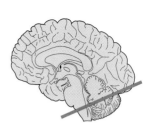

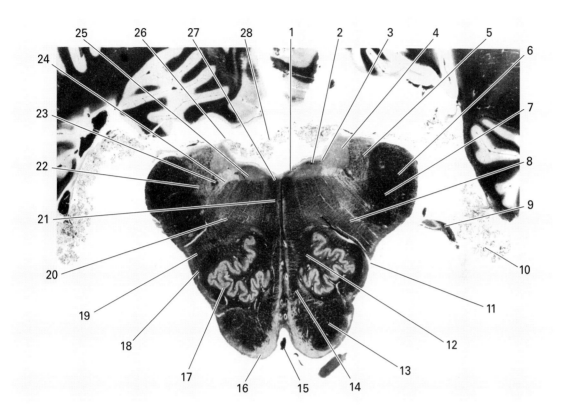

1	Internal arcuate fibers (striae medullares)
2	Posterior (dorsal) longitudinal fasciculus
3	Periventricular gray substance and limiting sulcus (sulcus limitans)
4	Medial vestibular nucleus (CN VIII)
5	Inferior vestibular nucleus (CN VIII)
6	Inferior cerebellar peduncle (restiform body)
7	Trigeminal nerve (CN V), spinal tract
8	Olivocerebellar tract
9	Vagus nerve (CN X), rootlet
10	Fourth ventricle (IV), lateral recess and choroid plexus
11	External arcuate fibers
12	Internal arcuate fibers
13	Corticospinal (pyramidal) tract
14	Medial lemniscus
15	Anterior spinal artery
16	Arcuate nucleus
17	Inferior olivary nucleus
18	Spinal lemniscus (spinoreticular, spinotectal, and spinothalamic tracts)
19	Rubrospinal tract
20	Medullary reticular formation (parvicellular nucleus)
21	Tectospinal tract
22	Trigeminal (CN V) spinal nucleus
23	Solitary tract
24	Solitary nucleus
25	Nucleus prepositus hypoglossi
26	Tenia choroidea
27	Medial longitudinal fasciculus
28	Choroid plexus and roof of fourth ventricle (IV)

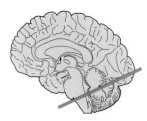

Transverse Section Through Glossopharyngeal Nerve Root (5X) with Vessel Territories

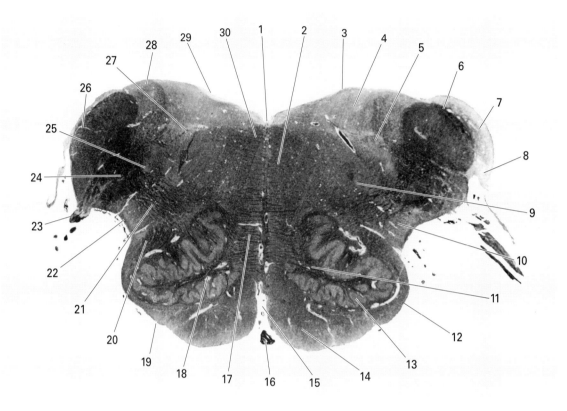

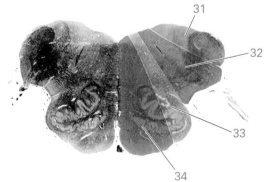

1	Median sulcus of fourth ventricle (IV)
2	Tectospinal tract
3	Medullary striae of fourth ventricle (IV)
4	Medial vestibular nucleus (CN VIII)
5	Solitary nucleus and tract
6	Dorsal acoustic stria
7	Posterior (dorsal) cochlear nucleus (CN VIII)
8	Posteroventral cochlear nucleus
9	Nucleus ambiguus (ventral motor nucleus of vagus nerve) (CN X)
10	Lateral reticular nucleus
11	Olivocerebellar fibers
12	Olivary eminence
13	Inferior olivary nucleus
14	Corticospinal (pyramidal) tract
15	Anterior (ventral) median fissure (sulcus)
16	Anterior spinal artery
17	Medial lemniscus
18	Inferior olive, (hilum)
19	External arcuate fibers
20	Spinal lemniscus (spinoreticular, spinotectal, and spinothalamic tracts)
21	Olivocerebellar tract (crossing fibers)
22	Anterior (ventral) spinocerebellar tract
23	Glossopharyngeal nerve root (IX)

24	Trigeminal nerve (CN V), spinal tract
25	Trigeminal (CN V) spinal nucleus
26	Inferior cerebellar peduncle, (restiform body)
27	Inferior salivatory nucleus
28	Inferior vestibular nucleus (CN VIII)
29	Limiting sulcus of fourth ventricle (IV), (sulcus limitans)
30	Medial longitudinal fasciculus
31	Anterior inferior cerebellar artery territory
32	Posterior inferior cerebellar artery territory
33	Vertebral artery territory
34	Anterior spinal artery territory

Transverse Section Through Vestibulocochlear Nerve Root (3X) with Vessel Territories

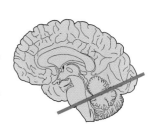

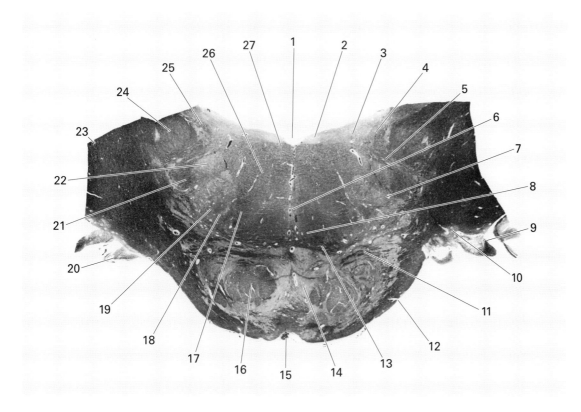

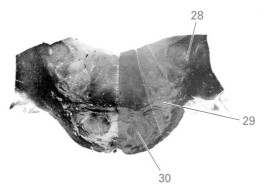

1	Median sulcus of fourth ventricle (IV)
2	Nucleus prepositus hypoglossi
3	Medial vestibular nucleus (CN VIII)
4	Lateral vestibular nucleus (CN VIII)
5	Vestibulocochlear nerve root (CN VIII)
6	Raphé nuclei
7	Facial nucleus (CN VII)
8	Medial lemniscus
9	Vestibulocochlear nerve (CN VIII)
10	Pontobulbar body
11	Pontocerebellar fibers
12	Middle cerebellar peduncle (brachium pontis)
13	Trapezoid body
14	Pontine nuclei (pontine gray)
15	Basilar sulcus of pons
16	Corticospinal (pyramidal) tract
17	Central tegmental tract
18	Superior olivary nucleus
19	Lateral lemniscus
20	Facial nerve rootlet (CN VII)
21	Trigeminal nerve (CN V), spinal tract
22	Trigeminal (CN V) spinal nucleus
23	Middle cerebellar peduncle (brachium pontis)
24	Inferior cerebellar peduncle (restiform body)
25	Vestibulocochlear nerve (CN VIII), descending branch

26	Pontine reticular formation (caudal part)
27	Medial longitudinal fasciculus
28	Anterior inferior cerebellar artery territory
29	Basilar artery, lateral branches territory
30	Basilar artery, medial branches territory

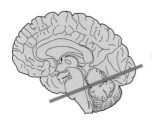

Transverse Section Through Facial Genu (3X)

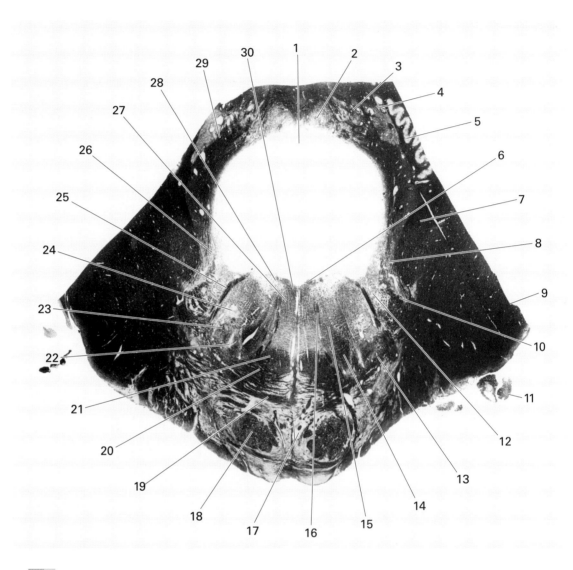

1	Fourth ventricle (IV)	16	Abducent nerve root (VI)
2	Fastigial nucleus	17	Pontine nuclei (pontine gray)
3	Globose nucleus	18	Corticospinal (pyramidal) tract
4	Emboliform nucleus	19	Pontocerebellar tract (crossing fibers)
5	Dentate nucleus	20	Trapezoid body
6	Facial nerve (CN VII), genu	21	Medial lemniscus
7	Inferior cerebellar peduncle (restiform body)	22	Superior olivary nucleus
8	Lateral vestibular nucleus (CN VIII)	23	Lateral lemniscus
9	Middle cerebellar peduncle (brachium pontis)	24	Facial nucleus (CN VII)
10	Trigeminal nerve (CN V), spinal tract	25	Facial nerve fibers (CN VII)
11	Trigeminal nerve (V)	26	Superior vestibular nucleus (CN VIII)
12	Trigeminal (CN V) spinal nucleus	27	Tectospinal tract
13	Spinal lemniscus (spinoreticular, spinotectal, and spinothalamic tracts)	28	Abducent nucleus (CN VI)
14	Central tegmental tract	29	Superior cerebellar peduncle (brachium conjunctivum)
15	Pontine reticular formation (inferior part)	30	Medial longitudinal fasciculus

Transverse Section Through Middle Pons (3X)

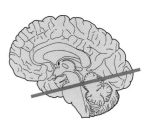

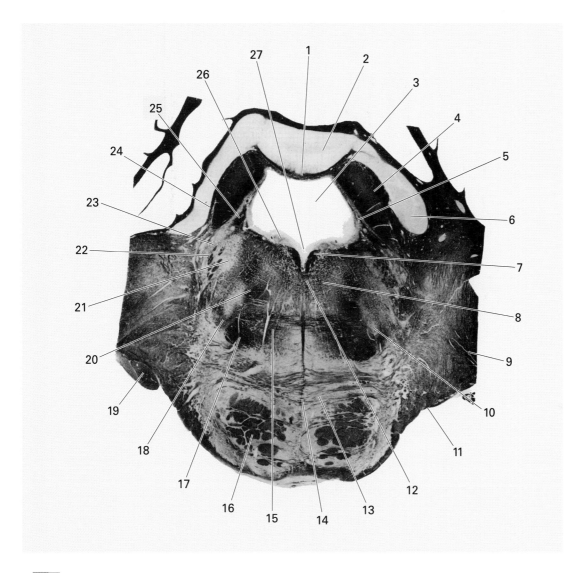

1	Superior medullary velum
2	Cerebellum, vermis, lingula
3	Fourth ventricle (IV)
4	Superior cerebellar peduncle (brachium conjunctivum)
5	Trigeminal (CN V) mesencephalic nucleus
6	Cerebellum, vermis, central lobule
7	Medial longitudinal fasciculus
8	Pontine reticular formation (superior part)
9	Middle cerebellar peduncle (brachium pontis)
10	Superior olivary nuclei and lateral lemniscus
11	Lateral pontine sulcus
12	Tectospinal tract
13	Pontine nuclei (pontine gray) and fibers
14	Raphé and pontocerebellar tract (crossing fibers)
15	Trapezoid body
16	Corticospinal (pyramidal) tract

17	Medial lemniscus
18	Lateral lemniscus
19	Trigeminal nerve (CN V)
20	Central tegmental tract
21	Trigeminal (CN V) motor nucleus
22	Trigeminal nerve root (CN V)
23	Trigeminal (CN V) main (principal) sensory nucleus
24	Anterior (ventral) spinocerebellar tract
25	Trigeminal nerve (CN V), mesencephalic tract
26	Posterior (dorsal) longitudinal fasciculus
27	Median sulcus of fourth ventricle (IV)

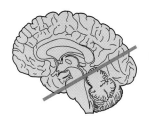

Transverse Section Through Superior Pons and Isthmus (4X)

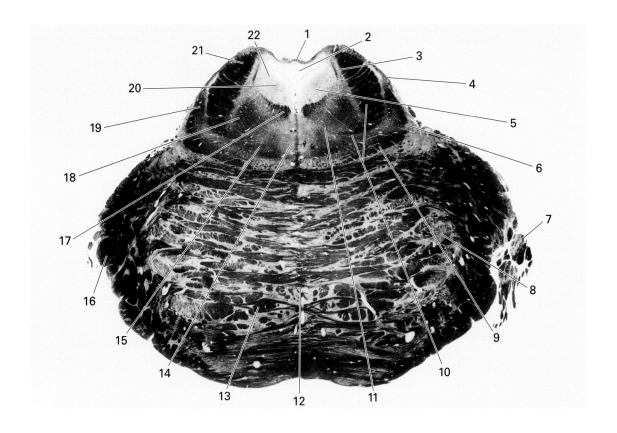

1 Superior medullary velum (decussation of anterior [ventral] spinocerebellar tract)
2 Fourth ventricle (IV)
3 Trigeminal nerve (CN V), mesencephalic tract
4 Anterior (ventral) spinocerebellar tract
5 Periaqueductal (central) gray substance
6 Spinal lemniscus (spinoreticular, spinotectal, and spinothalamic tracts)
7 Trigeminal nerve (CN V), root
8 Pontine nuclei (pontine gray)
9 Medial lemniscus
10 Superior cerebellar peduncle (brachium conjunctivum)
11 Pontine reticular formation (superior part)
12 Pontocerebellar tract (crossing fibers)
13 Corticospinal (pyramidal) tract
14 Raphé, central superior nucleus
15 Rubrospinal tract
16 Middle cerebellar peduncle (brachium pontis)
17 Medial longitudinal fasciculus
18 Central tegmental tract
19 Lateral lemniscus
20 Posterior (dorsal) longitudinal fasciculus
21 Superior cerebellar peduncle (brachium conjunctivum)
22 Locus ceruleus

Transverse Section Through Inferior Colliculus (4X) with Vessel Territories

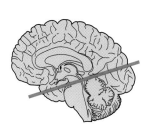

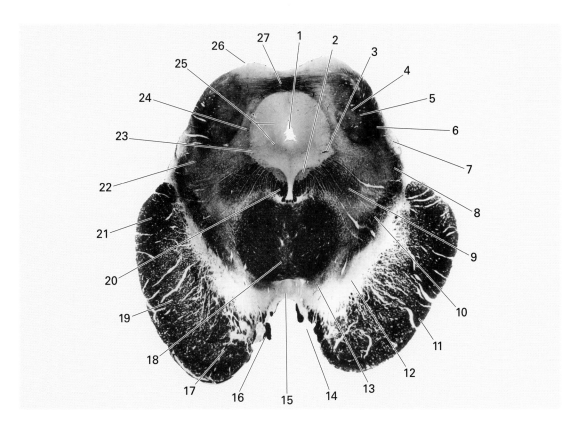

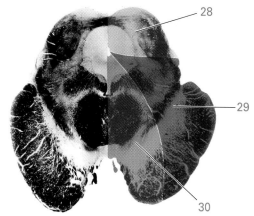

1	Cerebral aqueduct (aqueduct of *Sylvius*)
2	Trochlear nucleus (CN VI)
3	Midbrain tegmentum
4	Inferior colliculus, central nucleus
5	Inferior colliculus, brachium and external nucleus
6	Lateral lemniscus
7	Parabigeminal nucleus
8	Spinal lemniscus (spinoreticular, spinotectal, and spinothalamic tracts)
9	Central tegmental tract
10	Medial lemniscus
11	Cerebral peduncle
12	Substantia nigra
13	Mamillary peduncle
14	Interpeduncular fossa
15	Interpeduncular nucleus
16	Oculomotor nerve root (CN III)
17	Frontopontine tract
18	Decussation of superior cerebellar peduncles (brachia conjunctiva)
19	Corticospinal (pyramidal) and corticobulbar fibers
20	Medial longitudinal fasciculus
21	Temporopontine, occipitopontine, and parietopontine tracts
22	Reticular formation (cuneiform area)

23	Trigeminal nerve (CN V), mesencephalic nucleus
24	Trigeminal nerve (CN V), mesencephalic tract
25	Posterior (dorsal) longitudinal fasciculus (central gray substance)
26	Inferior colliculus
27	Commissure of inferior colliculus
28	Superior cerebellar artery territory
29	Posterior cerebral artery, collicular and posterior medial choroidal branches territory
30	Posterior cerebral artery, perforating branches territory

Transverse Section Through Oculomotor Nucleus (4X)

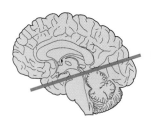

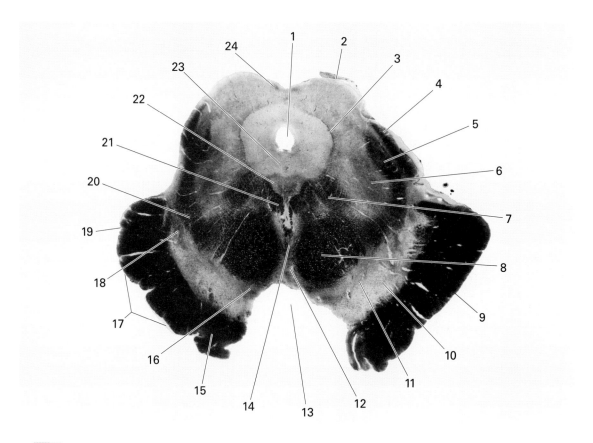

1	Cerebral aqueduct (aqueduct of *Sylvius*)
2	Superior colliculus
3	Trigeminal nerve (CN V), mesencephalic tract and nucleus
4	Inferior colliculus, brachium
5	Spinal lemniscus (spinoreticular, spinotectal, and spinothalamic tracts)
6	Reticular formation (cunieform nucleus)
7	Central tegmental tract
8	Superior cerebellar peduncle (brachium conjunctivum)
9	Cerebral peduncle
10	Substantia nigra, pars reticulata (reticular part)
11	Substantia nigra, pars compacta (compact part)
12	Anterior (ventral) tegmental decussation (crossing of rubrospinal tract)
13	Interpeduncular fossa
14	Posterior (dorsal) tegmental decussation (crossing of tectospinal tract)
15	Frontopontine tract
16	Mamillary peduncle
17	Corticospinal (pyramidal) and corticobulbar tracts
18	Pallidoreticular (lenticulonigral) tracts
19	Temporopontine, occipitopontine and parietopontine tracts
20	Medial lemniscus
21	Medial longitudinal fasciculus
22	Oculomotor nucleus (CN III)
23	Posterior (dorsal) longitudinal fasciculus and central gray substance
24	Commissure of superior colliculus

Transverse Section Through Superior Colliculus (3X) with Vessel Territories

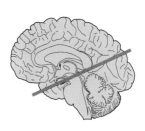

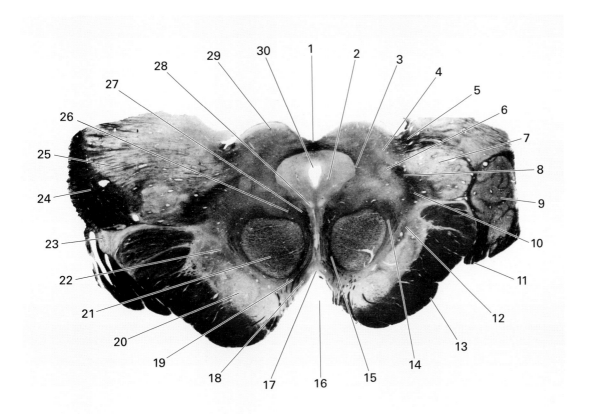

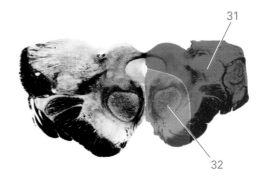

1	Posterior commissure and commissure of superior colliculus
2	Posterior (dorsal) longitudinal fasciculus
3	Trigeminal nerve (CN V), mesencephalic tract and nucleus
4	Pretectal area
5	Superior colliculus, brachium
6	Reticular formation (cunieform nucleus)
7	Thalamus, medial geniculate nucleus (MG) (medial geniculate body)
8	Spinothalamic tracts (anterior and lateral)
9	Thalamus, dorsal lateral geniculate nucleus (dLGN) (lateral geniculate body)
10	Medial lemniscus
11	Optic tract
12	Zona incerta
13	Cerebral peduncle
14	Superior cerebellar peduncle (brachium conjunctiuum)
15	Habenulo-interpeduncular tract (fasciculus retroflexus of *Meynert*)
16	Interpeduncular fossa
17	Ventral tegmental area
18	Mamillary peduncle
19	Oculomotor nerve root (CN III)
20	Substantia nigra

21	Red nucleus
22	Pallidoreticular (lenticulonigral) tracts
23	Thalamus, ventral lateral geniculate nucleus
24	Thalamus, external medullary lamina
25	Thalamus, pulvinar (Pul)
26	Central tegmental tract
27	Medial longitudinal fasciculus
28	Oculomotor (CN III) autonomic (*Edinger-Westphal*) nucleus
29	Superior colliculus
30	Cerebral aqueduct (aqueduct of *Sylvius*)
31	Posterior cerebral artery, collicular and posterior medial choroidal branches territory
32	Posterior cerebral artery, perforating branches territory

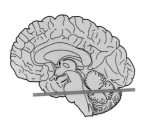

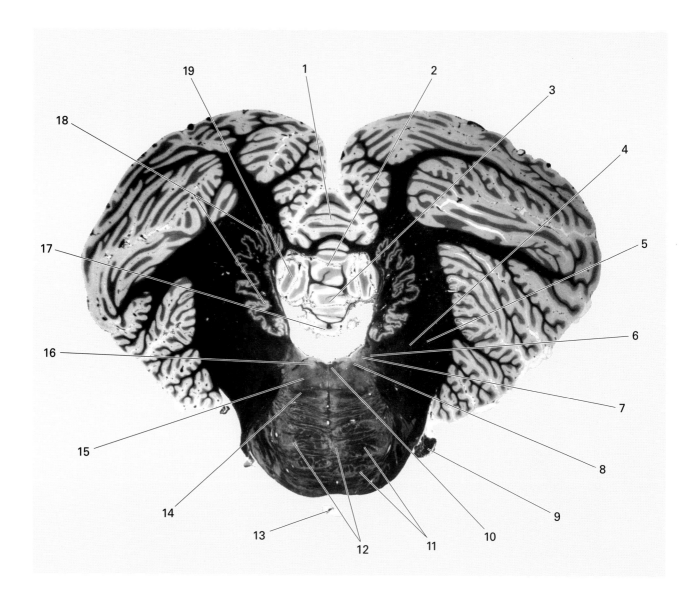

1	Tuber vermis
2	Cerebellum, vermis, pyramis
3	Cerebellum, vermis, uvula
4	Inferior cerebellar peduncle, (restiform body)
5	Middle cerebellar peduncle (brachium pontis)
6	Lateral vestibular nucleus (CN VIII)
7	Superior vestibular nucleus (CN VIII)
8	Facial nerve (CN VII)
9	Trigeminal nerve (CN V)
10	Medial longitudinal fasciculus

11	Corticospinal (pyramidal) and corticobular tracts
12	Pontine nuclei (pontine gray)
13	Basilar artery
14	Medial lemniscus
15	Central tegmental tract
16	Abducent nucleus (CN VI)
17	Cerebellum, vermis, nodule
18	Dentate nucleus
19	Cerebellum, tonsil (ventral paraflocculus)

Horizontal Section Through Fastigial Nucleus (1.5X)

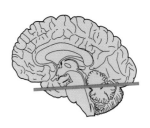

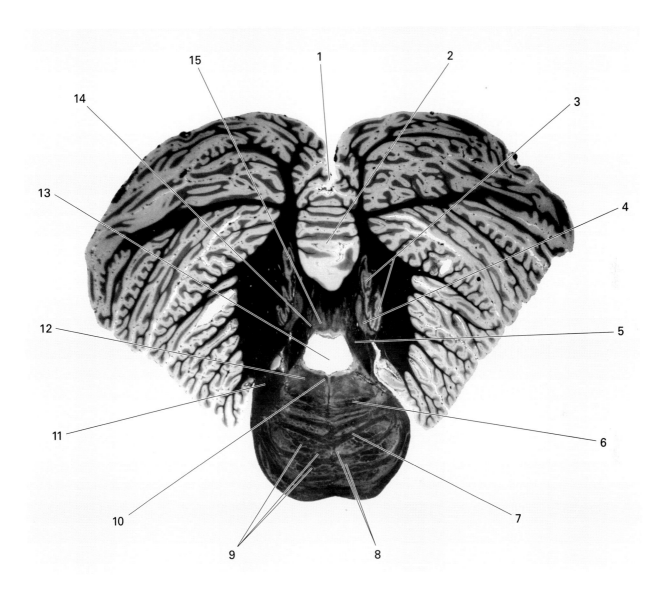

1	Cerebellum, folium vermis
2	Cerebellum, vermis, pyramis
3	Dentate nucleus
4	Emboliform nucleus
5	Superior cerebellar peduncle (brachium conjunctivum)
6	Medial lemniscus
7	Pontocerebellar fibers
8	Pontine nuclei (pontine gray)

9	Corticospinal (pyramidal) and corticobulbar tracts
10	Medial longitudinal fasciculus
11	Middle cerebellar peduncle (brachium pontis)
12	Central tegmental tract
13	Fourth ventricle (IV)
14	Globose nucleus
15	Fastigial nucleus

Histological Sections

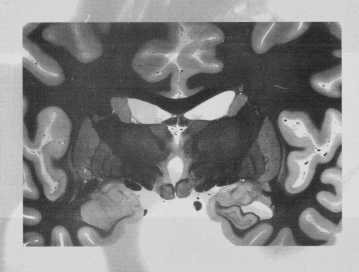

3. Basal Ganglia and Thalamus

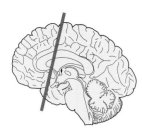

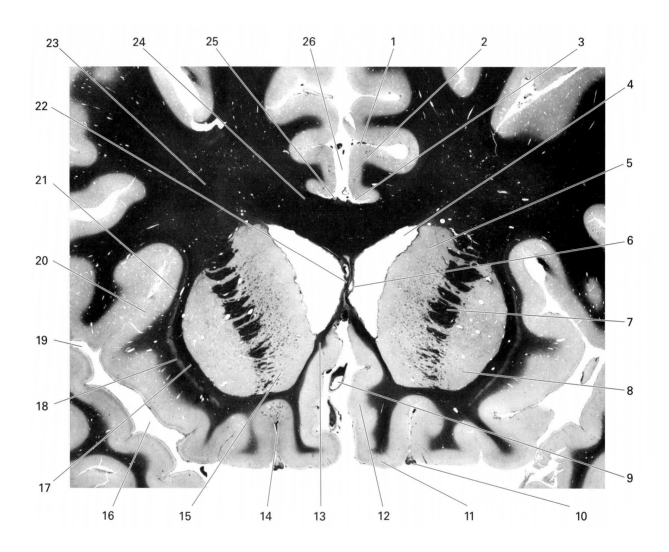

1	Cingulate sulcus	
2	Cingulate gyrus	
3	Callosal sulcus	
4	Lateral ventricle, frontal (anterior) horn	
5	Caudate nucleus, head	
6	Septal vein	
7	Internal capsule, anterior limb	
8	Putamen	
9	Anterior cerebral artery, pericallosal artery	
10	Olfactory tract	
11	Gyrus rectus (straight gyrus)	
12	Subcallosal area (gyrus)	
13	Corpus collosum, forceps minor	

14	Olfactory sulcus
15	Nucleus accumbens
16	Circular sulcus
17	External capsule
18	Claustrum
19	Lateral sulcus (*Sylvian* fissure)
20	Insula, short gyrus
21	Extreme capsule
22	Septum pellucidum
23	Corona radiata
24	Corpus callosum
25	Medial longitudinal stria (stria of *Lancisi*)
26	Longitudinal cerebral (interhemispheric) fissure

Coronal Section Through Optic Chiasm (1.5X)

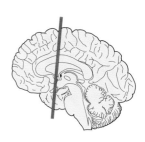

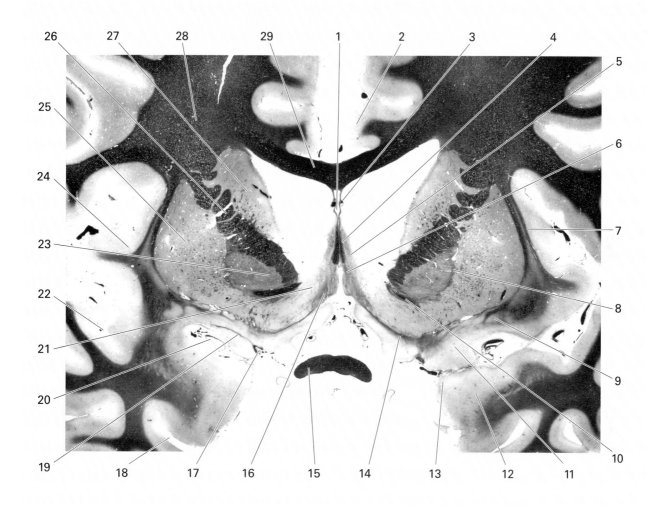

1 Septum pellucidum, cavum
2 Cingulate gyrus
3 Septal vein
4 Fornix, column
5 Septal nucleus
6 Vertical limb of diagonal band (diagonal band of *Broca*)
7 Claustrum
8 Globus pallidus, lateral medullary lamina
9 Claustrum, basal nuclei
10 Anterior commissure
11 Substantia innominata
12 Parahippocampal gyrus
13 Uncus
14 Horizontal limb of diagonal band (diagonal band of *Broca*)
15 Optic chiasm

16 Nucleus of diagonal band (gyrus, band of *Broca*)
17 Olfactory tract
18 Collateral sulcus
19 Lateral olfactory stria
20 Middle cerebral artery
21 Nucleus accumbens
22 Circular sulcus
23 Globus pallidus, internal (medial) segment (GPi)
24 Insular cortex
25 Putamen
26 Internal capsule, anterior limb
27 Caudate nucleus, head
28 Corona radiata
29 Corpus callosum

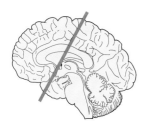

Coronal Section Through Anterior Commissure (1.5X)

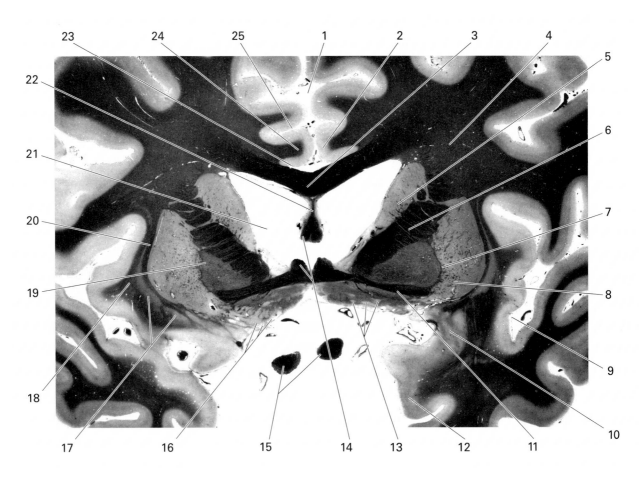

1	Longitudinal cerebral (interhemispheric) fissure
2	Cingulate gyrus
3	Corpus callosum
4	Corona radiata
5	Caudate nucleus, head
6	Internal capsule, anterior limb
7	Globus pallidus, lateral medullary lamina
8	Putamen
9	Insula, short gyri
10	Amygdala
11	Anterior commissure
12	Medial temporal cortex
13	Islands of *Calleja* (olfactory islets)
14	Fornix, column
15	Optic tract
16	Anterior perforated substance
17	Claustrum
18	Extreme capsule
19	Globus pallidus, external (lateral) segment (GPe)
20	External capsule
21	Lateral ventricle, frontal (anterior) horn
22	Septum pellucidum
23	Callosal sulcus
24	Cingulum
25	Cingulate sulcus

Coronal Section Through Anterior Thalamic Tubercle (1.5X)

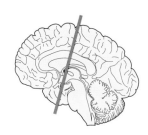

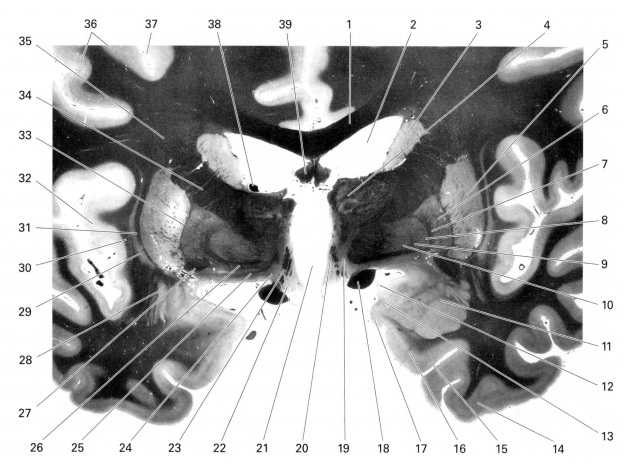

1	Corpus callosum	20	Hypothalamus, paraventricular nucleus
2	Lateral ventricle, body	21	Third ventricle (III)
3	Caudate nucleus, body	22	Hypothalamus, supraoptic nucleus
4	Thalamus, anterior nucleus (A)	23	Fornix, precommissural fibers
5	Putamen	24	Hypothalamus, supraoptic nucleus
6	Globus pallidus, external (lateral) segment (GPe)	25	Lateral olfactory stria
7	Globus pallidus, medial medullary lamina	26	Ansa lenticularis
8	Globus pallidus, internal (medial) segment (GPi), lateral part	27	Anterior commissure
		28	Amygdala, lateral nucleus
9	Globus pallidus, accessory medullary lamina	29	Claustrum
10	Globus pallidus, internal (medial) segment (GPi), medial part	30	Extreme capsule
		31	External capsule
11	Amygdala	32	Insular cortex
12	Semilunar gyrus	33	Globus pallidus, lateral medullary lamina
13	Semiannular sulcus	34	Internal capsule, genu
14	Lateral occipitotemporal gyrus	35	Corona radiata
15	Collateral sulcus	36	Middle frontal gyrus
16	Parahippocampal gyrus	37	Superior frontal sulcus
17	Uncus	38	Thalamostriate vein
18	Optic tract	39	Fornix, body
19	Lateral hypothalamic area		

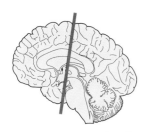

Coronal Section Through Mamillothalamic Tract (1.5X)

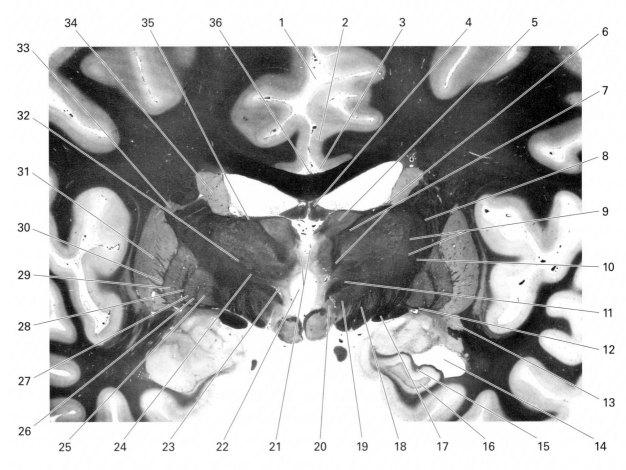

1	Longitudinal cerebral (interhemispheric) fissure
2	Cingulate gyrus
3	Callosal sulcus
4	Fornix, body
5	Thalamus, anterior nucleus (A)
6	Stria terminalis
7	Mamillothalamic tract
8	Thalamus, reticular nucleus
9	Thalamus, external medullary lamina
10	Internal capsule, posterior limb
11	Lenticular fasciculus (H$_2$ field of *Forel*)
12	Ansa lenticularis
13	Claustrum, basal nucleus
14	Lateral ventricle, temporal (inferior) horn
15	Hippocampus, alveus
16	Dentate gyrus
17	Optic tract
18	Substantia nigra
19	Subthalamic nucleus
20	Lateral hypothalamic area
21	Thalamus, midline nuclei
22	Third ventricle (III)
23	Hypothalamus, posterior nucleus
24	Thalamic fasciculus (H$_1$ field of *Forel*)
25	Globus pallidus, internal (medial) segment, (GPi), medial part
26	Globus pallidus, accessory medullary lamina
27	Globus pallidus, internal (medial) segment (GPi), lateral part
28	Globus pallidus, medial medullary lamina
29	Globus pallidus, external (lateral) segment (GPe)
30	Globus pallidus, lateral medullary lamina
31	Putamen
32	Thalamus, ventrolateral nucleus (VL)
33	Caudatolenticular gray bridges
34	Caudate nucleus, body
35	Thalamus, anterior radiations
36	Medial longitudinal stria (stria of *Lancisi*)

Coronal Section Through H Fields of *Forel* (1.5X)

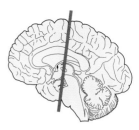

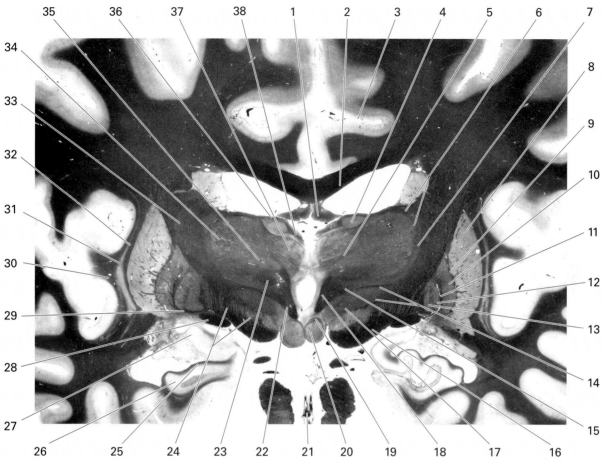

1	Fornix, body
2	Corpus callosum
3	Cingulate sulcus
4	Thalamus, laterodorsal nucleus (LD)
5	Thalamus, internal medullary lamina
6	Thalamus, external medullary lamina
7	Thalamus, reticular nucleus
8	Putamen
9	Globus pallidus, lateral medullary lamina
10	Globus pallidus, external (lateral) segment (GPe)
11	Globus pallidus, medial medullary lamina
12	Globus pallidus, internal (medial) segment (GPi), lateral part
13	Globus pallidus, internal (medial) segment (GPi), medial part
14	Subthalamic fasciculus
15	Zona incerta
16	Cerebral penuncle
17	Subthalamic nucleus
18	Mamillothalamic tract
19	Principal mamillary fasciculus
20	Mamillary body
21	Basilar artery
22	Lenticular fasciculus (H$_2$ field of *Forel*)
23	Thalamic fasciculus (H$_1$ field of *Forel*)
24	Substantia nigra
25	Hippocampus, alveus
26	Hippocampus
27	Amygdala
28	Optic tract
29	Ansa lenticularis
30	Extreme capsule
31	Claustrum
32	External capsule
33	Internal capsule, posterior limb
34	Thalamus, ventral posterolateral nucleus (VPL)
35	Thalamus, ventral posteromedial nucleus (VPM)
36	Thalamus, anterior radiations
37	Thalamus, dorsal medial nucleus (DM)
38	Stria medullaris of thalamus

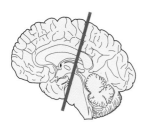

Coronal Section Through Dorsal Lateral Geniculate Nucleus (1.5X)

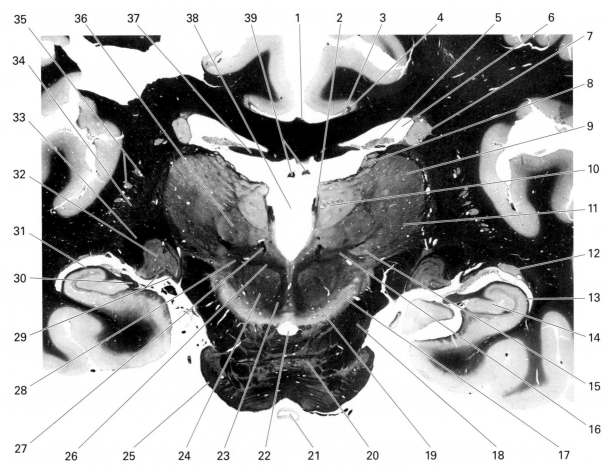

1	Medial longitudinal stria (stria of *Lancisi*)	22	Interpeduncular cistern
2	Stria medullaris of thalamus	23	Habenulo-interpeduncular tract (fasciculus retroflexus of *Meynert*)
3	Indusium griseum		
4	Lateral longitudinal stria (stria of *Lancisi*)	24	Red nucleus
5	Choroid plexus of lateral ventricle	25	Middle cerebellar peduncle (brachium pontis)
6	Lateral ventricle, trigone (atrium)	26	Mamillotegmental tract
7	Caudate nucleus, tail	27	Habenulo-interpeduncular tract (fasciculus retroflexus of *Meynert*)
8	Thalamus, laterodorsal nucleus (LD)		
9	Thalamus, lateroposterior nucleus (LP)	28	Dentatothalamic tract
10	Thalamus, dorsomedial nucleus (DM)	29	Optic tract
11	Thalamus, ventral posterolateral nucleus (VPL)	30	Hippocampus, fimbria
12	Caudate nucleus, tail	31	Hippocampus, alveus
13	Hippocampus	32	Thalamus, dorsal lateral geniculate nucleus (dLGN) (lateral geniculate body)
14	Dentate gyrus		
15	Thalamus, ventral posteromedial nucleus (VPM)	33	Optic radiations
16	Thalamus, ventral medial nucleus, posterior part	34	Internal capsule, posterior limb
17	Substantia nigra	35	Putamen
18	Cerebral peduncle	36	Thalamus, centromedian nucleus (CM)
19	Rubrospinal tract	37	Fornix, crus
20	Pontine nuclei (pontine gray)	38	Third ventricle (III)
21	Basilar artery	39	Internal cerebral veins

Coronal Section Through Pulvinar (1.5X)

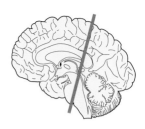

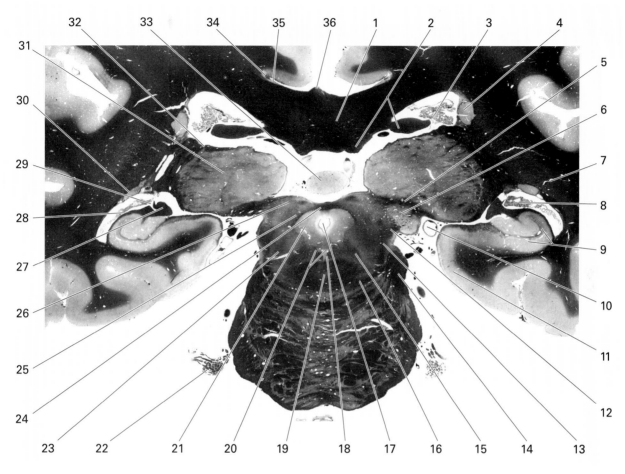

1	Corpus callosum, splenium
2	Fornix, crus
3	Choroid plexus (of lateral ventricle), glomus
4	Caudate nucleus, tail
5	Superior colliculus, brachium
6	Thalamus, medial geniculate nucleus (MG) (medial geniculate body)
7	Optic radiations
8	Choroid plexus of lateral ventricle, temporal (inferior) horn
9	Hippocampus
10	Posterior cerebral artery
11	Parahippocampal gyrus
12	Inferior colliculus, brachium
13	Spinothalamic tract (anterior and lateral)
14	Middle cerebellar peduncle (brachium pontis)
15	Central tegmental tract
16	Medial lemniscus
17	Cerebral aqueduct (aqueduct of *Sylvius*)

18	Medial longitudinal fasciculus
19	Superior cerebellar peduncle, decussation
20	Trochlear nuclei (CN IV)
21	Periaqueductal (central) gray substance
22	Trigeminal nerve (CN V)
23	Mesencephalic reticular formation
24	Posterior commissure
25	Trigeminal nerve (CN V), mesencephalic tract
26	Pretectal area
27	Hippocampus, fimbria
28	Hippocampus, alveus
29	Tenia of fimbria
30	Caudate nucleus, tail
31	Thalamus, pulvinar (Pul)
32	Thalamus, posterior peduncle
33	Pineal gland
34	Lateral longitudinal stria (stria of *Lancisi*)
35	Indusium griseum
36	Medial longitudinal stria (stria of *Lancisi*)

Histological Sections

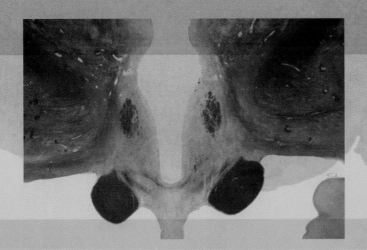

4. Hypothalamus, Basal Forebrain, and Hippocampus

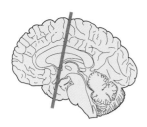

Coronal Section Through Optic Chiasm (5X)

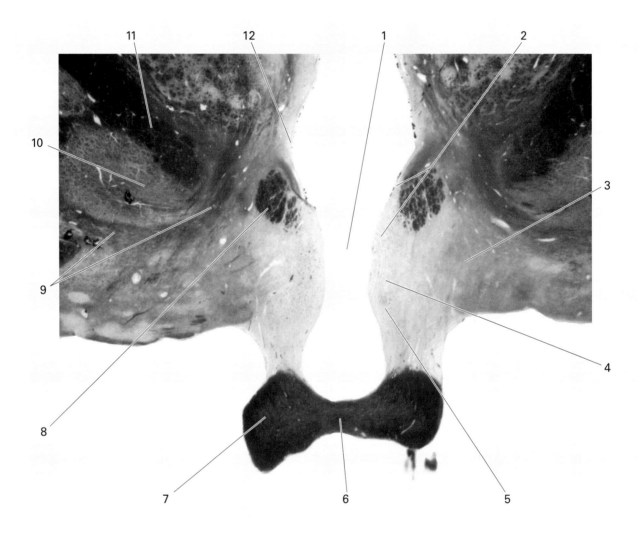

1	Third ventricle (III)
2	Hypothalamus, paraventricular nucleus
3	Lateral hypothalamic area
4	Hypothalamus, dorsomedial nucleus
5	Hypothalamus, ventromedial nucleus
6	Optic chiasm
7	Optic tract
8	Fornix, column
9	Ansa lenticularis
10	Globus pallidus, internal (medial) segment (GPi)
11	Internal capsule, posterior limb
12	Hypothalamic sulcus

Coronal Section Through Pituitary Stalk (5X)

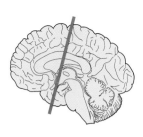

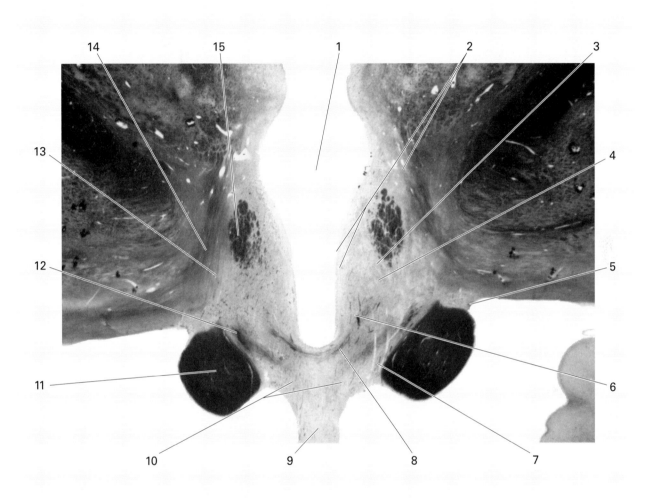

1	Third ventricle (III)
2	Hypothalamus, paraventricular nucleus
3	Hypothalamus, dorsomedial nucleus
4	Hypothalamus, ventromedial nucleus
5	Hypothalamus, supraoptic nucleus, dorsolateral part
6	Hypothalamus, anterior nucleus
7	Hypothalamus, supraoptic nucleus, ventromedial part
8	Dorsal supraoptic commissure
9	Infundibulum (pituitary stalk)
10	Hypothalamus, arcuate (infundibular) nuclei
11	Optic tract
12	Ventral supraoptic commissure
13	Lateral hypothalamic area and medial fore-brain bundle
14	Ansa lenticularis
15	Fornix, column

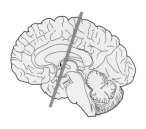

Coronal Section Through Interthalamic Adhesion (5X)

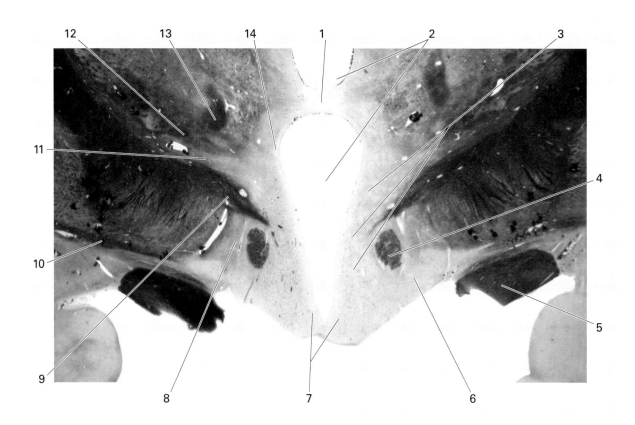

1	Interthalamic adhesion (massa intermedia)
2	Third ventricle (III)
3	Hypothalamus, posterior nucleus
4	Fornix, column
5	Optic tract
6	Hypothalamus, tuberomamillary nucleus
7	Hypothalamus, arcuate (infundibular) nuclei
8	Lateral hypothalamic area
9	Lenticular fasciculus (H$_2$ field of *Forel*)
10	Ansa lenticularis
11	Zona incerta
12	Thalamic fasciculus (H$_1$ field of *Forel*)
13	Mamillothalamic tract
14	Hypothalamic sulcus

Coronal Section Through Mamillary Bodies (5X)

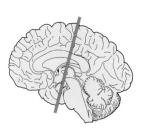

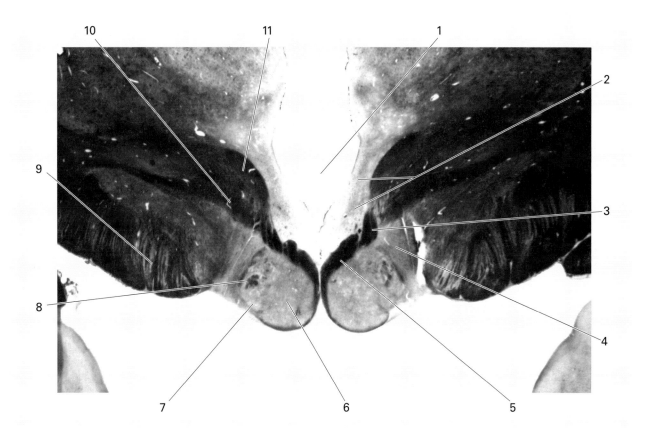

1	Third ventricle (III)
2	Hypothalamus, posterior nucleus
3	Mamillothalamic tract
4	Lateral hypothalamic area
5	Principal mamillary fasciculus
6	Hypothalamus, medial mamillary nucleus
7	Hypothalamus, lateral mamillary nucleus
8	Fornix, column
9	Substantia nigra
10	Lenticular fasciculus (H_2 field of *Forel*)
11	Thalamic fasciculus (H_1 field of *Forel*)

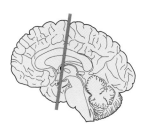

Coronal Section Through Olfactory Trigone and Nucleus Basalis (5X)

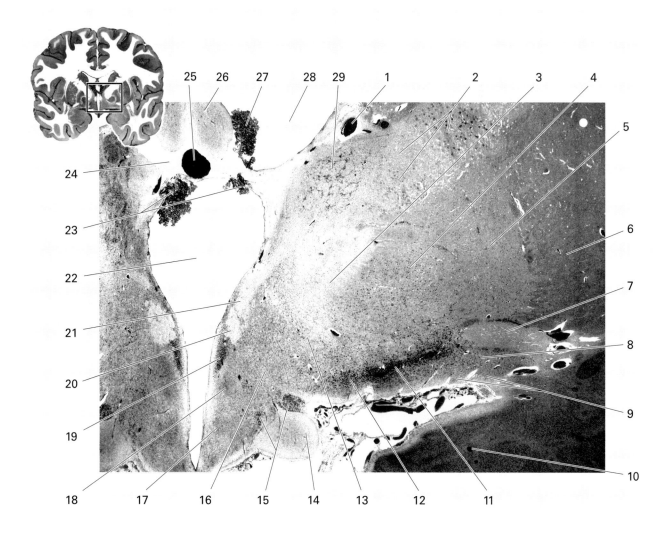

1	Thalamostriate vein
2	Internal Capsule
3	Ansa lenticularis
4	Globus pallidus, internal (medial) segment (GPi)
5	Globus pallidus, external (lateral) segment (GPe)
6	Putamen
7	Anterior commissure
8	Horizonal limb of diagonal band (diagonal band of *Broca*)
9	Anterior perforated substance
10	Amygdala and temporal lobe
11	Nucleus basalis (nucleus basalis of *Meynert*)
12	Substantia innominata
13	Inferior thalamic peduncle (radiations)
14	Optic tract
15	Hypothalamus, supraoptic nucleus
16	Lateral hypothalamic area
17	Hypothalamus, ventromedial nucleus
18	Hypothalamus, dorsomedial nucleus
19	Hypothalamus, paraventricular nucleus
20	Fornix, column
21	Stria medullaris of thalamus
22	Third ventricle (III)
23	Choroid plexus of third ventricle (III)
24	Velum interpositum
25	Internal cerebral vein
26	Fornix, body
27	Choroid plexus of lateral ventricle
28	Lateral ventricle
29	Thalamus, reticular nucleus

Coronal Section Through Body of Hippocampus (5X)

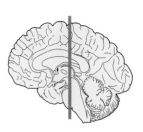

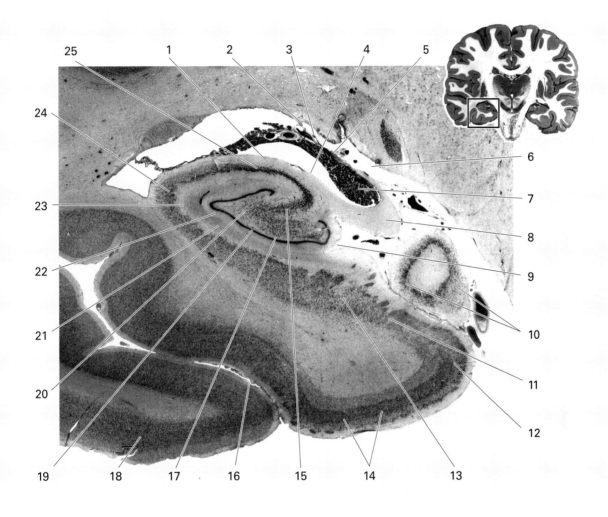

1	Hippocampus, stratum oriens	14	Parahippocampal gyrus
2	Tenia of stria terminalis	15	Hippocampus, CA3, pyramidal layer
3	Tela choroidea	16	Collateral sulcus
4	Hippocampus, alveus	17	Dentate gyrus, plexiform layer
5	Tenia of fimbria	18	Lateral occipitotemporal (fusiform) gyrus
6	Choroidal fissure	19	Dentate gyrus, granular layer
7	Choroid plexus	20	Dentate gyrus, polymorphic layer
8	Hippocampus, fimbria	21	Hippocampus, molecular layer
9	Hippocampal sulcus	22	Dentate gyrus, molecular layer
10	Intralimbic gyrus	23	Hippocampus, stratum radiatum
11	Presubiculum	24	Hippocampus, CA1, pyramidal layer
12	Parasubiculum	25	Hippocampus, CA2, pyramidal layer
13	Subiculum		

Pathways

Pathways

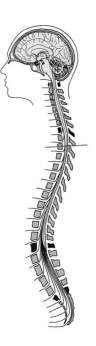

General Organization of Spinal Cord Gray Matter

The gray matter of the spinal cord is arranged as interrupted longitudinal columns separated into motor nuclei anteriorly and sensory nuclei posteriorly by the sulcus limitans.

Neural Tube
The neural tube has an anterior cell mass (**basal plate**—blue) that becomes the **anterior (ventral) horn** of the **spinal cord** and a posterior cell mass (**alar plate**—orange) that becomes the **posterior (dorsal) horn.** These are separated by the **sulcus limitans** of the **central canal. Somatic motor nuclei (SM**—red) and **visceral motor nuclei (VM**—violet) develop from the basal plate. **Visceral sensory (VS**—green) and **somatic sensory (SS**—blue) **nuclei** in the posterior (dorsal) horn develop from the alar plate. (The arrows indicate that the central canal opens at the fourth ventricle, page 179.)

Thoracic Spinal Cord
Embryonic patterns persist in the adult **spinal cord. Motor nuclei** for voluntary muscle (**SM**—red, to the **muscles** of the **abdominal wall**) are in the **anterior (ventral) horn,** and **preganglionic autonomic nuclei** for the viscera (**VM**—violet, to a **blood vessel**) are in the **lateral horn** or **intermediolateral cell column (nucleus).** Both nuclei are derived from the **basal plate.** Neurons in **visceral sensory (VS**—green, from a **blood vessel**) and **somatic sensory (SS**—blue, from the skin) **nuclei** are in the **posterior (dorsal) horn.** These nuclei are derived from the **alar plate.**

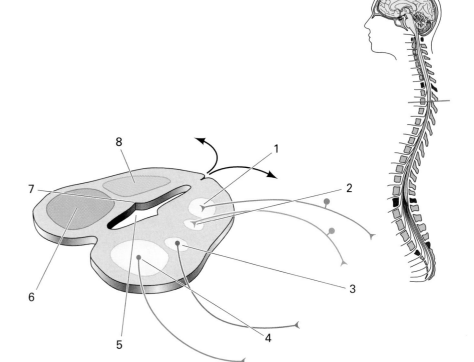

1	Somatic sensory nuclei (SS)
2	Visceral sensory nuclei (VS)
3	Visceral motor nuclei (VM)
4	Somatic motor nuclei (SM)
5	Central canal
6	Basal plate
7	Sulcus limitans
8	Alar plate

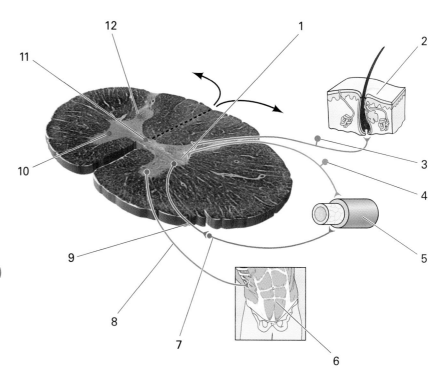

1	Lateral horn, intermediolateral cell column (nucleus)
2	Skin
3	Somatic afferent (posterior [dorsal] root ganglion cell)
4	Visceral afferent (posterior [dorsal] root ganglion cell)
5	Blood vessel
6	Abdominal muscle
7	Sympathetic neuron and fiber
8	Somatic efferent (motor neuron)
9	Visceral efferent (preganglionic neuron)
10	Basal plate (anterior [ventral] and lateral horns)
11	Sulcus limitans and central canal
12	Alar plate (posterior [dorsal] horn)

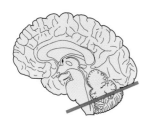

General Organization of Cranial Nerve Gray Matter

The gray matter of the brain stem, like that of the spinal cord, is arranged as interrupted longitudinal columns separated into motor nuclei medially and sensory nuclei laterally by the sulcus limitans.

Brain stem

The plan of the neural tube is preserved in the brain stem, where the central canal opens posteriorly to form the **fourth ventricle (IV). Motor** and **sensory cranial nerve nuclei** related to the **basal** and **alar plates,** respectively, are separated by the **sulcus limitans.** To the elements found in the **spinal cord** are added motor nuclei related to muscles of the head and neck that develop in the branchial arches, **branchiomotor nuclei (BM—** mustard), and nuclei that receive inputs from the ear, **special sensory nuclei (SPS—pink).**

Open Medulla

In the open medulla (page 184), cranial nerve nuclear columns are related to features on the floor of the **fourth ventricle (IV).** The **sulcus limitans** separates motor columns derived from the **basal plate** (blue) medially and sensory columns derived from the **alar plate** (orange) laterally. Nuclei of the motor columns in this section, from medial to lateral, are **somatic motor (SM—**red, **hypoglossal nucleus, CN XII** to the **tongue), branchiomotor (BM—mustard, nucleus ambiguus, CN X** to the **larynx),** and **visceral motor (VM—**violet, **dorsal motor nucleus, CN X** to a **blood vessel).** The sensory columns, from medial to lateral, are **visceral sensory (VS—**green, **nucleus of the solitary tract, CN X** from a **blood vessel), somatic sensory (SS—**blue, **trigeminal [CN V] spinal nucleus, CN V** from the **skin** of the head and neck), and **special sensory (SPS—**pink, **descending** and **medial vestibular nuclei [CN VIII], hair cells** in the labyrinth).

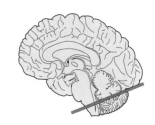

1	Fourth ventricle (IV)
2	Special sensory nuclei (SPS)
3	Visceral sensory nuclei (VS)
4	Somatic sensory nuclei (SS)
5	Branchiomotor nuclei (BM)
6	Visceral motor nuclei (VM)
7	Pyramid (corticospinal tract)
8	Inferior olivary nucleus
9	Somatic motor nuclei (SM)
10	Basal plate
11	Alar plate
12	Sulcus limitans

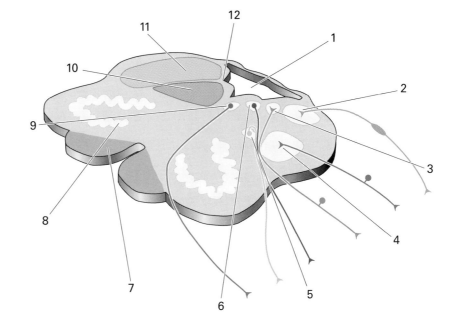

1	Hypoglossal nucleus (CN XII)
2	Fourth ventricle (IV)
3	Dorsal motor nucleus (CN X)
4	Solitary nucleus
5	Descending and medial vestibular nuclei (CN VIII)
6	Vestibulocochlear nerve (CN VIII)
7	Vestibular hair cell
8	Skin
9	Trigeminal (CN V) spinal nucleus
10	Somatic afferent (trigeminal ganglion cell)
11	Visceral afferent (nodose ganglion cell)
12	Blood vessel
13	Parasympathetic ganglion cell
14	Branchiomotor efferent
15	Laryngeal muscles
16	Visceral efferent (preganglionic neuron)
17	Tongue muscles
18	Somatic motor efferent
19	Nucleus ambiguus (CN X)
20	Pyramid (corticospinal tract)
21	Inferior olivary nucleus
22	Basal plate
23	Alar plate
24	Sulcus limitans

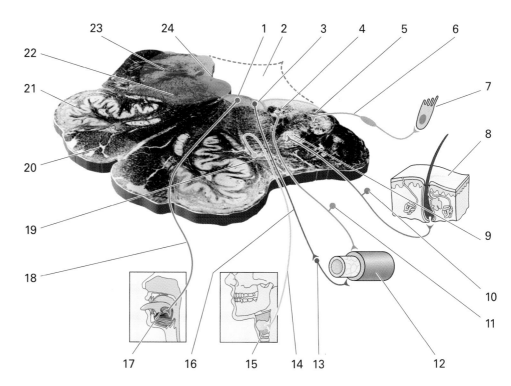

Sensory Cranial Nerves and Nuclei

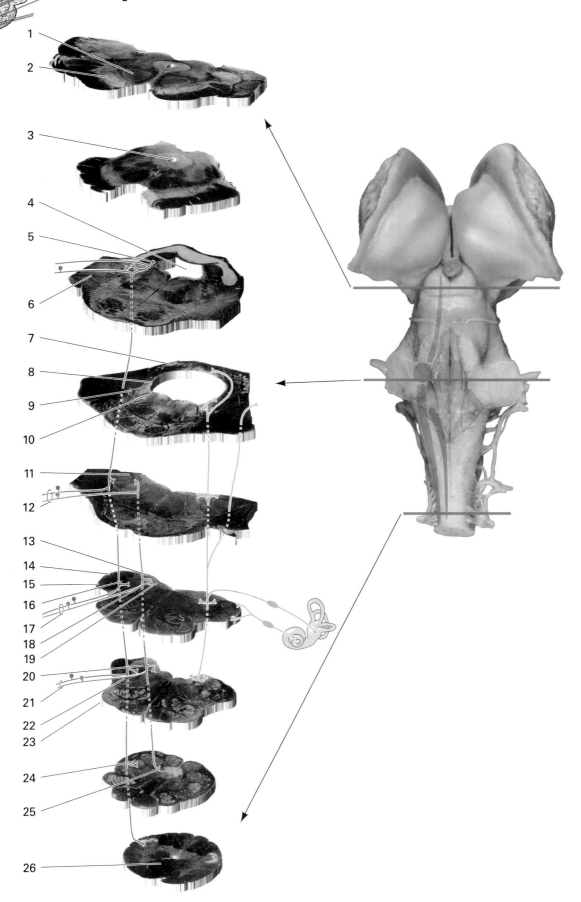

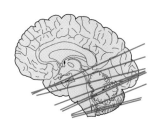

1. Red nucleus
2. Substantia nigra
3. Cerebral aqueduct (aqueduct of *Sylvius*)
4. Fourth ventricle (IV)
5. Trigeminal nerve (CN V), mesencephalic nucleus
6. Trigeminal nerve (CN V)
7. Dentate nucleus
8. Superior vestibular nucleus (CN VIII)
9. Trigeminal (CN V) main (principal) sensory nucleus
10. Facial nerve (CN VII), genu
11. Lateral vestibular nucleus (CN VIII)
12. Facial nerve (CN VII)
13. Inferior vestibular nucleus (CN VIII)
14. Posterior (dorsal) cochlear nucleus (CN VIII)
15. Anterior (ventral) cochlear nucleus (CN VIII)
16. Trigeminal (CN V, VII, IX, X) spinal nucleus
17. Glossopharyngeal nerve (CN IX)
18. Solitary nucleus (CN VII, IX)
19. Medial vestibular nucleus (CN VIII)
20. Solitary nucleus (CN VII, IX, X)
21. Vagus nerve (CN X)
22. Trigeminal (CN V, VII, IX, X) spinal nucleus
23. Inferior olive
24. Trigeminal (CN V, VII, IX, X) spinal nucleus
25. Solitary nucleus (CN VII, IX, X)
26. Pyramidal decussation (corticospinal tracts)

Neurons in the brain stem sensory nuclei are arranged in continuous columns similar to the sensory areas of the posterior horn of the spinal cord.

The **visceral sensory column (VS**—green) the **solitary nucleus**—receives fibers from the **facial nerve (CN VII)** for taste on the anterior two thirds of the tongue, the **glossopharyngeal nerve (CN IX)** for taste on the posterior third of the tongue, and the **vagus nerve (CN X)** for taste buds in the pharynx. All project to the superior half of the nucleus. The inferior portion of the nucleus receives sensory fibers mainly through the **vagus nerve (CN X)** from the heart, lungs, blood vessels, and GI tract. The **somatic sensory column (SS**—blue) receives inputs from the **trigeminal (CN V), facial (CN VII), glossopharyngeal (CN IX),** and **vagus (CN X) nerves**. These fibers innervate structures that develop from the branchial arches in the head, neck, oral and nasal cavities, and upper pharynx. All pain from the head, face, and neck carried by these nerves is relayed through the **trigeminal (CN V) spinal nucleus;** fine touch is relayed through the trigeminal (CN V) spinal nucleus and the **main sensory trigeminal nucleus.** Vibration and position sense are carried by primary afferent neurons in the **mesencephalic nucleus** of the **trigeminal nerve (CN V). The special sensory column (SPS**—pink) and the vestibular and auditory relay nuclei of the **vestibulocochlear nerve (CN VIII)** receive fibers from the vestibular apparatus (saccule, utricle, and semicircular canals) and the cochlea.

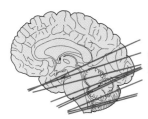

Motor Cranial Nerves and Nuclei

The motor nuclei related to different classes of targets (muscles from somites and branchial arches and muscles and glands in viscera) are in separated interrupted longitudinal columns.

The **somatic motor nuclei (SM**—red) are a superior continuation of the motor neuron pools of the anterior horn of the spinal cord. This column consists of the **hypoglossal nucleus (CN XII)** controlling muscles of the tongue and nuclei controlling muscles that move the eye, namely, the **abducent nucleus (CN VI)** supplying the **lateral rectus muscle**; the **trochlear nucleus (CN III)** supplying the **superior oblique muscle**; and the **oculomotor nucleus (CN III)** supplying the **medial, inferior,** and **superior rectus muscles** and the **inferior oblique muscle**. The **branchiomotor nuclei (BM**—blue) supply muscles derived from the branchial arches. This column consists of the **trigeminal (CN V) motor nucleus** supplying **muscles** of **mastication, digastric** and **mylohyoid muscles,** and **tensors** of the **palate** and the **ear drum**; the **facial nucleus (CN VII)** supplying **muscles** of **facial expression** above and below the eyes; the **platysma, buccinator,** and **stapedius muscles**; and the **nucleus ambiguus,** which contributes to the **glossopharyngeal (IX), vagus (CN X),** and **accessory (CN IX) nerves** to innervate the **stylopharyngeus,** the **superior** and **middle pharyngeal constrictors,** the **laryngeal muscles,** and all **muscles** of the **palate** except the tensor; the **spinal accessory motor nucleus (CN IX)** gives rise to fibers to the **sternomastoid** and **upper trapezius** muscles. The **visceromotor nuclei (VM**—green) in the midbrain, pons, and medulla are the cranial division of the parasympathetic system. The **autonomic nuclei** of the **oculomotor nucleus (CN III)** (*Edinger-Westphal* nucleus) supplies the **ciliary ganglion,** innervating the **ciliary body** and **iris** to regulate the curvature of the lens and the diameter of the pupil; the **superior salivatory nucleus** of the **facial nerve (CN VII)** supplies ganglia to regulate secretions of the **lacrimal, sublingual,** and **submaxillary glands**; the **inferior salivatory nucleus** through the **glossopharyngeal nerve (CN IX)** regulates secretions from the **parotid gland**; and the **dorsal motor nucleus** of the **vagus nerve (CN X)** supplies glands for secre-

tions in the **pharynx, airways (trachea and bronchi), lungs,** and **GI tract** to the splenic flexure; the conducting system of the **heart**; and peripheral ganglia that regulate smooth muscle tone in **blood vessels, lungs,** and **GI tract.**

1	Oculomotor nucleus (CN III), autonomic nuclei (*Edinger-Westphal* nucleus)
2	Oculomotor nucleus (CN III)
3	Oculomotor nerve (CN III)
4	Trochlear nerve (CN IV)
5	Trochlear nucleus (CN IV)
6	Trigeminal (CN V) motor nucleus
7	Trigeminal nerve (CN V)
8	Abducent nucleus (CN VI)
9	Facial nerve (CN VII), motor nucleus
10	Abducent nerve (CN VI)
11	Facial nerve (CN VII)
12	Superior salivatory nucleus (CN VII)
13	Facial nerve (CN VII)
14	Inferior salivatory nucleus (CN IX)
15	Nucleus ambiguus (ventral motor nucleus of vagus nerve) (CN IX)
16	Glossopharyngeal nerve (CN IX)
17	Dorsal (posterior) nucleus of vagus nerve (CN X)
18	Nucleus ambiguus (ventral motor nucleus of vagus nerve) (CN X)
19	Vagus nerve (CN X)
20	Dorsal (posterior) nucleus of vagus nerve (CN X)
21	Hypoglossal nucleus (CN XII)
22	Nucleus ambiguus (ventral motor nucleus of vagus nerve) (CN X)
23	Vagus nerve (CN X)
24	Hypoglossal nerve (CN XII)
25	Accessory nerve (CN XI)
26	Accessory nucleus (CN XI)

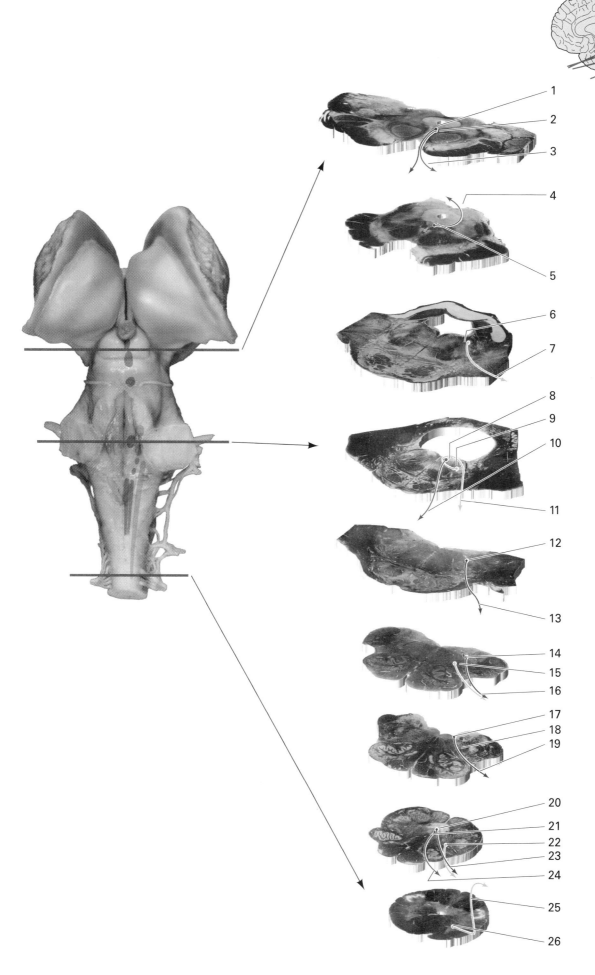

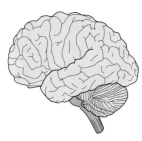

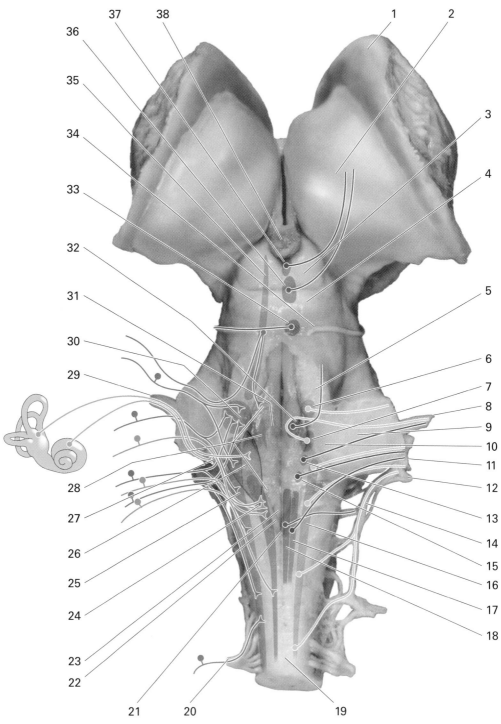

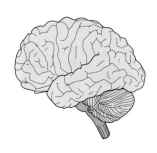

1 Caudate nucleus
2 Thalamus
3 Superior colliculus
4 Inferior colliculus
5 Superior cerebellar peduncle
(brachium conjunctivum)
6 Trigeminal (CN V) motor nucleus
7 Facial nucleus (CN VII)
8 Facial nerve (CN VII)
9 Middle cerebellar peduncle (brachium pontis)
10 Inferior cerebellar peduncle (restiform body)
11 Glossopharyngeal and vagus nerves (CN IX, X)
12 Accessory nerve (CN XI)
13 Superior salivatory nucleus (CN VII)
14 Accessory nerve (CN XI) spinal root
15 Inferior salivatory nucleus (CN IX)
16 Nucleus ambiguus and spinal accessory nucleus (CN IX, X, XI)
17 Dorsal (posterior) nucleus of vagus nerve (CN X)
18 Hypoglossal nucleus (CN XII)
19 Spinal cord
20 Spinal nerve (C2), posterior (dorsal) root (ramus)
21 Obex
22 Vagal (CN X) trigone
23 Hypoglossal (CN XII) trigone
24 Solitary nucleus (CN VII, IX, X)
25 Trigeminal (CN V, VII, IX, X) spinal nucleus
26 Vestibular nuclei (CN VIII)
27 Cochlear nuclei (CN VIII)
28 Sulcus limitans
29 Vestibulocochlear nerve (CN VIII)
30 Trigeminal (CN V) main (principal) sensory nucleus
31 Facial colliculus
32 Abducent nucleus (CN VI)
33 Trochlear nucleus (CN IV)
34 Trochlear nerve (CN IV)
35 Trigeminal (CN V) mesencephalic nucleus
36 Oculomotor nucleus (CN III)
37 Oculomotor nucleus (CN III), autonomic nuclei
(*Edinger-Westphal* nucleus)
38 Pineal gland

The nuclei of the cranial nerves are arranged as interrupted longitudinal columns through the length of the brain stem, separated into motor nuclei medially and sensory nuclei laterally by the sulcus limitans.

The posterior (dorsal) aspect of the **brain stem** with projections of the cranial nerve nuclei and cranial nerves is shown. The **sulcus limitans** on the floor of the fourth ventricle grossly separates **motor columns** medially from **sensory columns** laterally. The association of the cranial nerves with their nuclei is best appreciated from the anterior (ventral) aspect of the brain stem (page 187).

The motor nuclear columns are, medial to lateral: a) **somatic motor column (SM**—red, **CN III, IV, VI, XII);** b) **branchiomotor column (BM**—mustard, **CN V, VII, IX, X, IX);** and c) **visceral motor column (VM**—violet, **CN III, VII, IX, X).**

The sensory nuclear columns are, medial to lateral: a) **visceral sensory column (VS**—green, **CN VII, IX, X);** b) **somatic sensory (SS**—blue, **CN V, VII, IX, X);** and **special sensory (SPS**—pink, **CN VIII).**

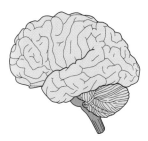

Organization of Cranial Nerve Nuclei into Columns–Anterior Aspect

The nuclei of the cranial nerves are arranged as interrupted longitudinal columns through the length of the brain stem, separated into motor nuclei medially and sensory nuclei laterally.

The association of the cranial nerves with their nuclei is best appreciated from the anterior (ventral) aspect of the brain stem.
The **sulcus limitans** on the floor of the fourth ventricle grossly separates **motor columns** medially from **sensory columns** laterally. The posterior (dorsal) aspect of the brain stem with projections of the cranial nerve nuclei and cranial nerves is shown on page 184.

The motor nuclear columns are, medial to lateral: a) **somatic motor column (SM**—red, **CN III, IV, VI, XII)**; b) **branchiomotor column (BM**—mustard, **CN V, VII, IX, XI)**; and c) **visceral motor column (VM**—violet, **CN III, VII, IX, X)**.

The sensory nuclear columns are, medial to lateral: a) **visceral sensory column (VS**—green, **CN VII, IX, X)**; b) **somatic sensory (SS**—blue, **CN V, VII, IX, X)**; and **special sensory (SPS**—pink, **CN VIII)**.

1	Optic chiasm
2	Oculomotor nucleus (CN III), autonomic nuclei (*Edinger-Westphal* nucleus)
3	Olfactory tract
4	Optic nerve (CN II)
5	Optic tract
6	Trochlear nerve (CN IV)
7	Cerebral peduncle
8	Trigeminal nerve (CN V)
9	Trigeminal (CN V) mesencephalic nucleus
10	Trigeminal (CN V) main (principal) sensory nucleus
11	Vestibulocochlear nerve (CN VIII)
12	Cochlear nuclei (CN VIII)
13	Glossopharyngeal nerve (CN IX)
14	Vagus nerve (CN X)
15	Vestibular nuclei (CN VIII)
16	Accessory nerve (CN XI)
17	Solitary nucleus (CN VII, IX, X)
18	Trigeminal (CN V, VII, IX, X) spinal nucleus
19	Spinal nerve (C2)
20	Anterior (ventral) median fissure (sulcus)
21	Hypoglossal nucleus (CN XII)
22	Spinal accessory nucleus (CN XI)
23	Nucleus ambiguus (CN IX, X, XI)
24	Spinal nerve (C1)
25	Dorsal (posterior) nucleus of vagus nerve (CN X)
26	Inferior salivatory nucleus (CN IX)
27	Superior salivatory nucleus (CN VII)
28	Facial nerve (CN VII), motor nucleus
29	Hypoglossal nerve (CN XII)
30	Abducent nucleus (CN VI)
31	Facial nerve (CN VII)
32	Abducent nerve (CN VI)
33	Trigeminal (CN V) motor nucleus
34	Pons
35	Trochlear nucleus (CN IV)
36	Oculomotor nerve (CN III)
37	Oculomotor nucleus (CN III)
38	Caudate nucleus

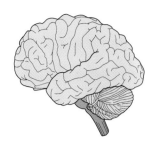

1

2 3 4

38

37

5

36

6

35

7

34

8

33

9

32

10

31

11

30

12
13

29

28

14

27

15

26

16

25 24 23 22 21 20 19

17

18

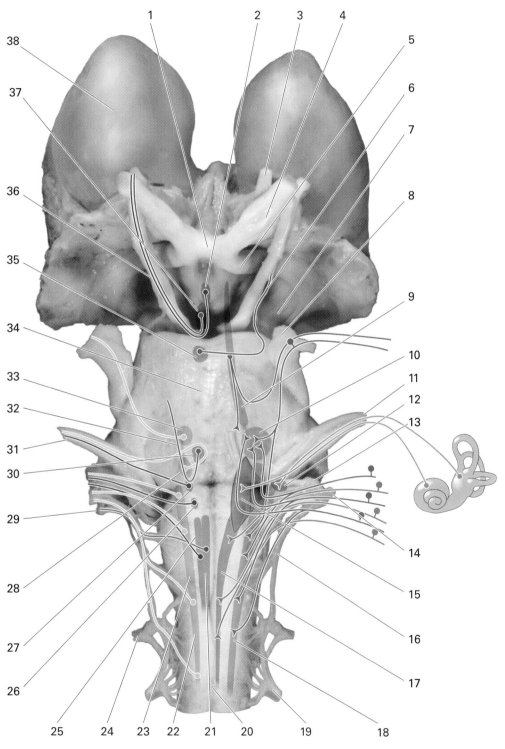

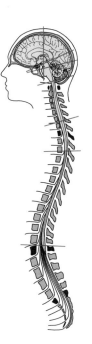

Touch and Position Sense Pathways: Posterior (Dorsal) Column/Medial Lemniscus and Trigeminal Main Sensory Nucleus

This pathway carries fine discriminative and active touch, body and joint position, and vibration sense.

Myelinated and heavily myelinated **spinal nerve axons**—the **first-order neurons**—from **posterior (dorsal) root ganglion** cells enter the medial aspect of the **posterior (dorsal) root entry zone** of the **spinal cord.** They ascend to the brain stem in the **posterior (dorsal) columns** with sacral fibers closer to the midline and cervical fibers closer to the dorsal horn. The first synapse is in the **posterior (dorsal) column nuclei** of the **caudal medulla:** lumbosacral fibers in the **gracile fasciculus** and **nucleus** and thoracocervical fibers in the **cuneate fasciculus** and **nucleus.** Cranial nerve axons from the head, mainly from the **trigeminal (CN V) nerve** but also from the **facial (CN VII), glossopharyngeal (CN IX),** and **vagus (CN X) nerves,** enter the brain stem laterally. The first synapse is in the **trigeminal (CN V) main (principal) sensory nucleus** in the **pons** (pages 180 and 184). **Second-order axons** from the posterior (dorsal) column nuclei cross in the ventral medulla to form the **medial lemniscus,** which ascends on the opposite side, with sacral fibers ventral and upper thoracic fibers dorsal. In the **pons,** the **medial lemniscus** rotates from a parasagittal to a transverse orientation so that sacral fibers are lateral and cervical fibers are medial. These are joined on their medial aspect by fibers from the **trigeminal (CN V) main (principal) sensory nucleus** of the opposite side. In the lateral **midbrain tegmentum,** the **medial lemniscus** rotates farther, with sacral fibers dorsolateral and trigeminal fibers ventromedial, prior to terminating in the **ventral posterolateral (VPL)** and **ventral posteromedial (VPM) nuclei** of the **thalamus.** From the thalamus, **third-order axons** ascend in the **internal capsule, posterior limb,** to terminate in the **somatosensory cortex** of the **postcentral gyrus** and **parietal operculum** (*Brodmann's* areas **1, 2,** and **3b**) of the **parietal lobe.**

1   Parietal lobe
2   Corpus callosum
3   Internal capsule, posterior limb
4   Lateral sulcus (*Sylvian* fissure)
5   Thalamus, ventral posterolateral (VPL) and ventral
     posteromedial (VPM) nuclei
6   Midbrain tegmentum
7   Red nucleus
8   Fourth ventricle (IV)
9   Trigeminal (CN V) main (principal) sensory nucleus
10   Pons
11   Medial lemniscus
12   Gracile fasciculus and nucleus
13   Cuneate fasciculus and nucleus
14   Pyramids (corticospinal tracts)
15   Posterior (dorsal) root entry zone
16   Posterior (dorsal) root ganglion
17   Posterior (dorsal) columns
18   Spinal cord
19   Spinal nerve
20   Anterior (ventral) horn

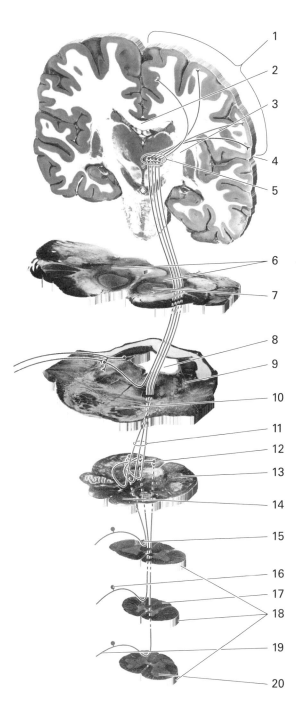

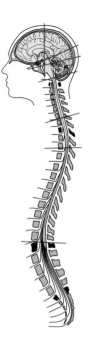

Touch Pathways: Anterior and Lateral Spinothalamic Tracts and Trigeminal Spinal Nucleus

This system carries the sensations of pain, temperature, and crude and fine touch.

Myelinated, finely myelinated, and unmyelinated **spinal nerve axons** innervating the body from **posterior (dorsal) root** and **cranial nerve root ganglion** cells enter the **spinal cord** and **brain stem** through the lateral **posterior (dorsal) root** and **cranial nerve root entry zones.** In the spinal cord, they terminate on neurons in the **posterior (dorsal) horn** at the spinal segment of entry. Myelinated, finely myelinated, and unmyelinated fibers innervating the head, face, and mouth from **trigeminal (CN V), facial (CN VII), glossopharyngeal (CN IX),** and **vagal (CN X) ganglion cells** enter the brain stem to join the trigeminal spinal tract and synapse on neurons in the **trigeminal (CN V) spinal nucleus** (pages 184 and 187). **Second-order axons** cross in the **anterior white commissure** to ascend in the contralateral **lateral funiculus.** These fibers form a distinct tract in the lateral **medulla,** where they are joined by axons from the opposite **trigeminal (CN V) spinal nucleus,** which cross in the medulla. Fibers are ordered: those conveying sensation from the leg are layered parallel to and superficial to those from the chest and arm, which are superficial to those from the head. In the **midbrain,** spinothalamic fibers are posterior and lateral to the **lateral lemniscus** prior to terminating in the **ventral posterolateral (VPL)** and **ventral posteromedial (VPM) nuclei** of the **thalamus.** In the thalamus there is a topographic pattern with the legs lateral and the trunk, arms, hands, and face medial. **Third-order axons** from the thalamus ascend in the **posterior limb** of the **internal capsule** to end in cortex of the **postcentral gyrus** and **parietal operculum (***Brodmann's* **areas 1, 2,** and **3a)** of the **parietal lobe.**

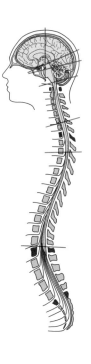

1	Parietal lobe
2	Thalamus, ventral posterolateral nucleus (VPL)
3	Thalamus, ventral posteromedial nucleus (VPM)
4	Internal capsule, posterior limb
5	Substantia nigra
6	Central canal
7	Thalamus, medial geniculate nucleus (MG) (medial geniculate body)
8	Red nucleus
9	Cerebral peduncle
10	Superior cerebellar peduncle (brachium conjunctivum)
11	Lateral lemniscus
12	Medial lemniscus
13	Trigeminal (CN V) spinal nucleus
14	Inferior olive
15	Spinal nerve
16	Posterior (dorsal) horn
17	Posterior (dorsal) root ganglion
18	Lateral funiculus
19	Posterior (dorsal) root entry zone
20	Anterior white commissure

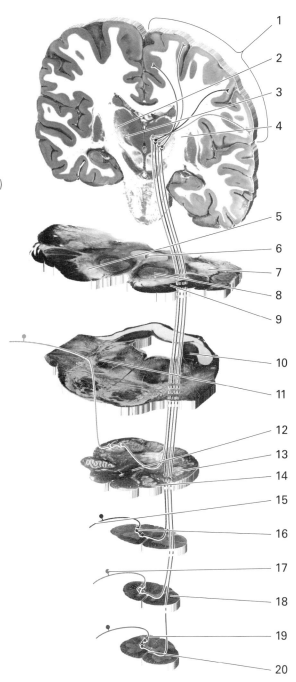

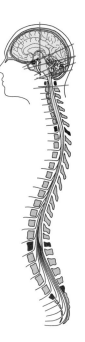

Touch Pathways: Head and Face

This system transmits fine and crude touch and pain and temperature information from the head, face, mouth, and pharynx.

Axons arise from **first-order neurons** in the **trigeminal (CN V) ganglion** and enter the **pons** via the **trigeminal nerve root (CN V)** to terminate in the **trigeminal (CN V) main (principal) sensory nucleus** for touch and the **trigeminal (CN V) spinal nucleus** for touch, pain, and temperature. Somatic sensory inputs from neurons in the **facial (geniculate) (CN VII)**, **superior** and **inferior (petrosal) glossopharyngeal (CN IX)**, and **superior (jugular)** and **inferior (nodose) vagal (CN X) ganglia** also project to these nuclei (pages 184 and 187). Fibers in the **trigeminal nerve (CN V) sensory root** for fine touch take a direct medial course to the main sensory nucleus. Trigeminal fibers to the spinal nucleus descend in the **spinal tract** of the **trigeminal nerve (CN V)** through the lateral **pontine tegmentum** and the **lateral medulla** to the **substantia gelatinosa** of the **posterior (dorsal) horn** of the upper cervical **spinal cord.** The fibers terminate in different locations: those from the lower part of the face (V3, mandibular division of the trigeminal nerve) project mainly to the rostral pontine part, those from the midface (V2, maxillary division) to the medullary part, and those from the upper face (V1, ophthalmic division) to the spinal part. The **trigeminal (CN V) mesencephalic nucleus** contains first-order neurons (ganglion cells that migrated into the central nervous system during development). Position sense is carried in peripheral axons of neurons in the mesencephalic nucleus that enter the pons at the lateral angle of the **fourth ventricle (IV)** and ascend as the **trigeminal nerve (CN V) mesencephalic tract,** which lies adjacent to the fourth ventricle and medial to the **superior cerebellar peduncle.** The central axons of these cells terminate on neurons in the **trigeminal (CN V) motor nucleus** and the **trigeminal main** and **spinal nuclei.**

Most **second-order axons** from the **trigeminal main sensory** and **spinal nuclei** cross to the opposite side just superior to these nuclei. A smaller uncrossed component represents somatic structures near the midline. Axons from the spinal nucleus are just medial to the **spinothalamic tracts (anterior and lateral)** as they ascend posterior to the **inferior olivary nucleus** in the medulla. In the **pontine** and **midbrain tegmentum,** fibers from the main sensory nucleus join the medial aspect of the **medial lemniscus.** Fibers from the main sensory and spinal nuclei end in the **ventral posteromedial nucleus (VPM)** of the **thalamus.** From there, fibers project to the **postcentral gyrus** and the **parietal operculum** (*Brodmann's* **areas 3b, 1,** and **2**).

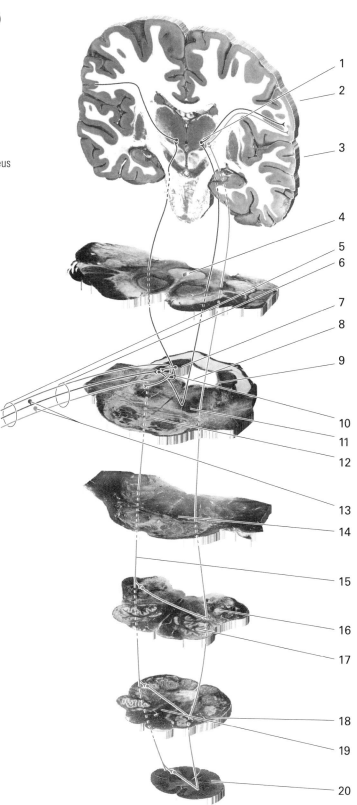

1 Thalamus, ventral posteromedial nucleus (VPM)
2 Parietal operculum
3 Temporal lobe
4 Cerebral aqueduct (aqueduct of *Sylvius*)
5 Trigeminal nerve (CN V)
6 Trigeminal nerve root (CN V)
7 Trigeminal (CN V) mesencephalic nucleus
8 Fourth ventricle (IV)
9 Trigeminal nerve (CN V), mesencephalic tract
10 Trigeminal (CN V) main (principal) sensory nucleus
11 Medial lemniscus
12 Pons
13 Trigeminal (CN V) ganglion
14 Trapezoid body
15 Trigeminal nerve (CN V), spinal tract
16 Trigeminal (CN V, VII, IX, X) spinal nucleus
17 Inferior olivary nucleus
18 Spinothalamic tracts (anterior and lateral)
19 Medial lemniscus
20 Substantia gelatinosa (posterior [dorsal] horn)

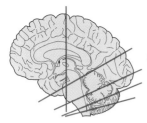

Taste Pathways

These pathways carry taste sensation from receptors on the surface of the tongue, pharynx, and soft palate.

This is a crossed and ipsilateral pathway. **First-order axons** of ganglion cells of the **facial (CN VII), glossopharyngeal (CN IX)**, and **vagus (CN X) nerves** enter the rostral lateral **medulla** and pass via the ipsilateral **solitary tract** to the superior, gustatory part of the **solitary nucleus. Second-order axons** ascend ipsilaterally in the **solitary fasciculus** to terminate in the **medial parabrachial nucleus** of the **midbrain tegmentum. Third-order axons** ascend on the same side or cross with trigeminal fibers to the medial part of the **ventral posteromedial nucleus (VPMm)** of the **thalamus. Fourth-order axons** from the thalamus project via the **posterior limb** of the **internal capsule** to the **frontoparietal operculum** (a forward extension of *Brodmann*'s **areas 3b** and **3a).**

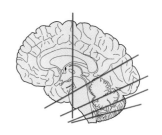

1 Longitudinal cerebral (interhemispheric) fissure
2 Thalamus, ventral posteromedial nucleus (VPMm), medial part
3 Frontal and parietal opercula
4 Internal capsule, posterior limb
5 Hippocampus
6 Superior cerebellar peduncle (brachium conjunctivum)
7 Parabrachial nucleus
8 Middle cerebellar peduncle (brachium pontis)
9 Corticospinal (pyramidal) tract
10 Facial nerve (CN VII)
11 Taste afferents
12 Solitary fasciculus
13 Glossopharyngeal nerve (CN IX)
14 Solitary nucleus (CN VII, IX, X)
15 Solitary tract
16 Inferior cerebellar peduncle (restiform body)
17 Vagus nerve (CN X)
18 Gracile fasciculus and nucleus
19 Trigeminal (CN V) spinal nucleus
20 Pyramid (corticospinal tract)

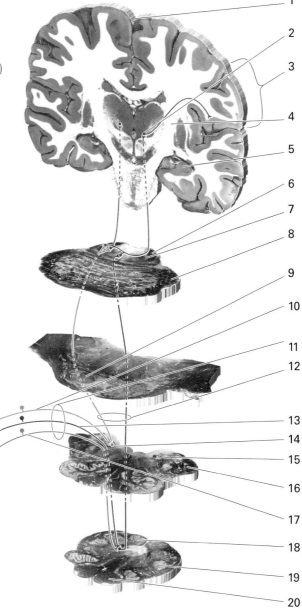

1
2
3
4
5
6
7
8
9
10
11
12
13
14
15
16
17
18
19
20

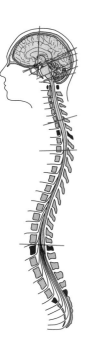

Autonomic Pathways: Afferents

These pathways carry information to the brain from the pelvic viscera, gastrointestinal tract, lungs, heart, blood vessels, and other internal organs of the abdomen, thorax, neck, and head.

Small myelinated and unmyelinated fibers from the **viscera** in **spinal roots** and the **vagus (CN X)** and **trigeminal nerves (CN V)** project to the **inferior part** of the **nucleus** of the **solitary tract**. This nucleus projects alongside the **spinal lemniscus** to the **lateral parabrachial nucleus** and **periaqueductal gray substance** of the **midbrain**, where the fibers join the **medial forebrain bundle** on their way to the **lateral hypothalamic area**, the **paraventricular nucleus** of the **hypothalamus**, the **central nucleus** of the **amygdala**, and the **interstitial nucleus** of the **stria terminalis.** The inferior solitary nucleus also projects extensively throughout the medulla and pons, notably to nuclei projecting to **parasympathetic ganglia** (page 201).

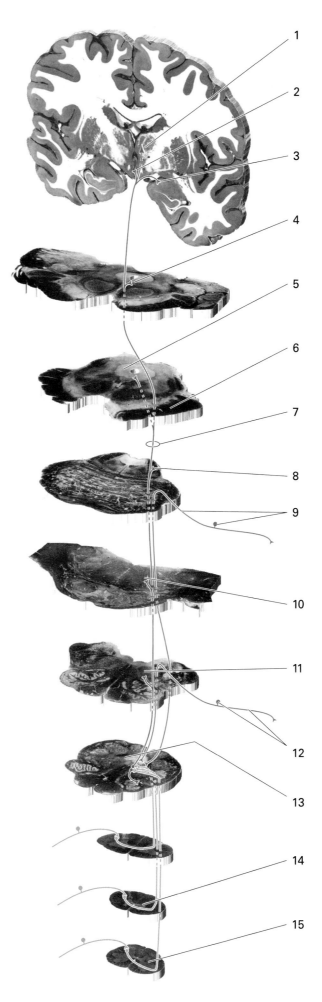
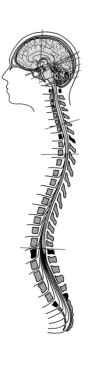

1 Fibers to stria terminalis, interstitial nucleus
2 Hypothalamus, paraventricular nucleus and lateral hypothalamic area, and medial forebrain bundle
3 Amygdala, central nucleus
4 Oculomotor nucleus (CN III), autonomic nuclei (*Edinger-Westphal* nucleus)
5 Periaqueductal (central) gray substance
6 Cerebral peduncle
7 Ascending fibers from solitary nucleus (CN VII, IX, X), inferior part
8 Lateral parabrachial nucleus
9 Trigeminal root and ganglion (CN V)
10 Superior salivatory nucleus (CN VII)
11 Inferior salivatory nucleus (CN IX)
12 Vagus nerve (CN X) and ganglion, inferior (nodose)
13 Solitary nucleus (CN VII, IX, X), inferior part
14 Lateral horn, intermediolateral cell column (nucleus)
15 Lateral horn, intermediolateral cell column (nucleus)

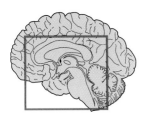

Autonomic Pathways: Sympathetic Efferents

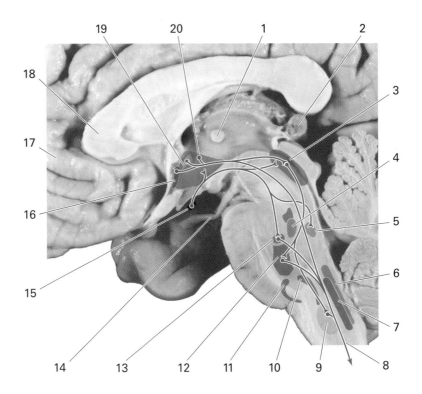

These pathways control responses to external and internal stimuli such as increased heart rate and blood pressure, bronchodilation, decreased gastrointestinal motility and secretion, and sweating and piloerection, which together occur as the "fight or flight" response to emergencies.

Descending sympathetic fibers in the **brain stem** and the **spinal cord** arise from the **paraventricular** and **medial preoptic nuclei** of the **hypothalamus**, the **lateral hypothalamic area**, the **central nucleus** of the **amygdala**, and several cell groups in the **inferior medulla**.

The fibers from the **hypothalamus** and **amygdala** split in the upper **midbrain** to form a medial pathway via the **dorsal longitudinal fasciculus** under the floor of the **fourth ventricle (IV)** and a lateral pathway via the **anterolateral tegmentum**, ultimately emerging posterolateral to the **inferior olive** to descend in the posterior part of the **lateral fasciculus** of the **spinal cord** as the **hypothalamospinal tract**.

Fibers from the **hypothalamus** and **amygdala** are joined by axons from the **A5 cell group**, the lateral parts of the **reticular formation** in the **medulla,** and the **raphé nucleus magnus,** which project to the **intermediolateral cell column** of **lateral horn** in the **thoracic spinal cord** via the **hypothalamospinal tract.** Preganglionic fibers from the **lateral horn** exit the **spinal cord** to innervate the nearby **paravertebral** and **preaortic sympathetic ganglia.** These neurons innervate blood vessels, sweat glands, piloerector muscles, pupils, heart, lungs, gastrointestinal tract, and all other viscera.

1	Interthalamic adhesion (massa intermedia)
2	Pineal gland
3	Periaqueductal (central) gray substance
4	Barrington's nucleus
5	Parabrachial nuclei
6	Solitary nucleus (CN VII, IX, X)
7	Dorsal (posterior) nucleus of vagus nerve (CN X)
8	Hypothalamospinal tract
9	Reticular formation, medulla
10	Raphé nucleus obscurus
11	Raphé nucleus pallidus
12	Raphé nucleus magnus
13	A5 cell group
14	Oculomotor nerve (CN III)
15	Amygdala, central nucleus
16	Hypothalamus, medial preoptic nucleus
17	Cingulate gyrus
18	Corpus callosum, genu
19	Hypothalamus, paraventricular nucleus
20	Hypothalamus, lateral area
21	Hypothalamus
22	Temporal lobe
23	Thalamus, dorsal lateral geniculate nucleus (dLGN) (lateral geniculate body)
24	Posterior (dorsal) longitudinal fasciculus
25	Cerebral aqueduct (aqueduct of *Sylvius*)
26	Substantia nigra
27	Cerebral peduncle
28	Central tegmental tract
29	Middle cerebellar peduncle (brachium pontis)
30	Superior salivatory nucleus (CN VII)
31	Dorsal (posterior) nucleus of vagus nerve (CN X)
32	Inferior cerebellar peduncle (restiform body)
33	Hypoglossal nucleus (CN XII)
34	Central canal
35	Lateral funiculus
36	Lateral horn, intermediolateral cell column (nucleus)
37	Sympathetic ganglion neuron
38	Anterior (ventral) horn

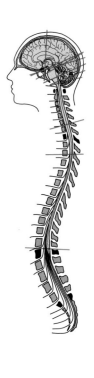

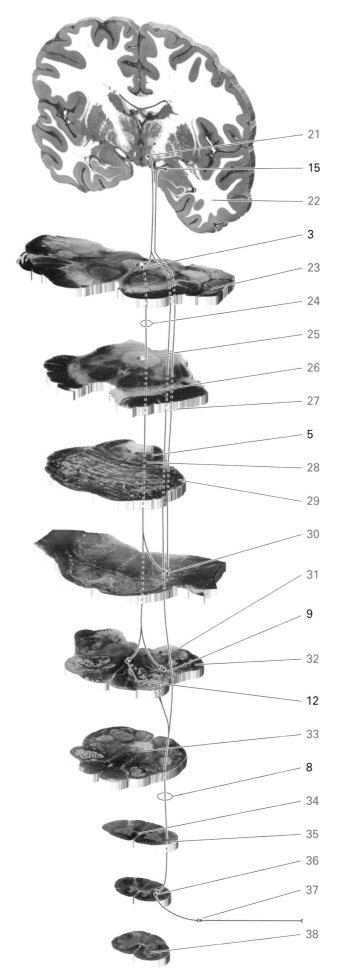

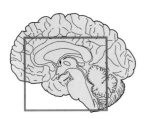

Autonomic Pathways: Parasympathetic Efferents

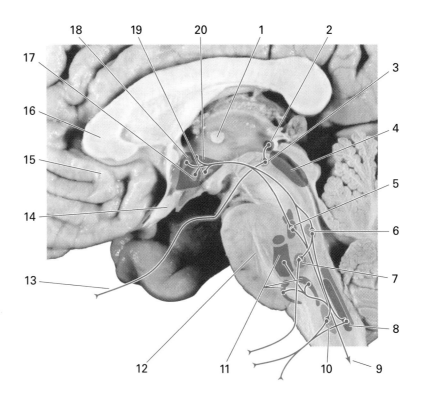

These pathways control responses to external and internal stimuli such as pupillary constriction, accommodation of the lens, tearing, salivation, heart rate, gastrointestinal motility and secretion, erection, defecation, and micturition.

Descending fibers to the **brain stem** and the **spinal cord** arise from the **cingulate gyrus** of the cerebral cortex; the **paraventricular, posterior,** and **dorsomedial nuclei** of the **hypothalamus;** the **lateral hypothalamic area;** and several nuclei in the **pons** and **medulla.**

The main targets of these axons are the **medial parabrachial nucleus,** which, in turn, projects to the parasympathetic cranial nerve nuclei of the **superior (CN VII)** and **inferior (CN IX) salivatory nuclei;** the **dorsal (posterior) nucleus** of the **vagus nerve (CN X);** and around the **nucleus ambiguus (ventral motor nucleus** of **vagus nerve) (CN X)** and the nearby **Barrington's nucleus.** The principal inputs to the *Edinger-Westphal*

nucleus are from the **pretectal area,** which receives direct projections from the **eyes.** Axons from **Barrington's nucleus** are joined by fibers from the **raphé nuclei (magnus, obscurus,** and **pallidus)** to project to preganglionic parasympathetic neurons in the **lateral horn** of the **sacral spinal cord** via the **hypothalamospinal tract.**

The **parasympathetic nervous system** is divided into **cranial** and **sacral divisions.** Peripheral targets of the cranial division are the **ciliary (CN III), pterygopalatine (CN VII), submandibular (CN VII),** and **otic (CN IX) ganglia** in the head and neck and **parasympathetic ganglion cells** in the viscera of the neck, thorax, and abdomen (**CN X,** heart and gut to the splenic flexure of the colon). Targets of the sacral division (via motor roots of spinal nerves S2-S4) are ganglion cells in the viscera of the lower abdomen and pelvis (descending colon, rectum, urinary bladder, and sexual organs).

1	Interthalamic adhesion (massa intermedia)
2	Pretectal area
3	Oculomotor nucleus (CN III), autonomic nuclei (*Edinger-Westphal* nucleus)
4	Periaqueductal (central) gray substance
5	Barrington's nucleus
6	Parabrachial nuclei
7	Superior and inferior salivatory nuclei (CN VII, IX)
8	Dorsal (posterior) nucleus of vagus nerve (CN X)
9	Hypothalamospinal tract
10	Nucleus ambiguus (ventral motor nucleus of vagus nerve) (CN X)
11	Raphé nuclei magnus, obscurus, and pallidus
12	Pons
13	Oculomotor nerve (CN III)
14	Optic chiasm
15	Cingulate gyrus
16	Corpus callosum, genu
17	Hypothalamus, dorsomedial nucleus
18	Hypothalamus, paraventricular nucleus
19	Hypothalamus, posterior nucleus
20	Hypothalamus, lateral area
21	Hypothalamus
22	Temporal lobe
23	Ciliary ganglion
24	Substantia nigra
25	Middle cerebellar peduncle (brachium pontis)
26	Dorsal longitudinal fasciculus
27	Lateral vestibular nucleus (CN VIII)
28	Facial nerve (CN VII)
29	Pterygopalatine, submandibular, and otic ganglia
30	Hypoglossal nucleus (CN XII)
31	Vagus nerve (CN X) and ganglion cell
32	Lateral funiculus
33	Anterior (ventral) horn
34	Lateral horn, intermediolateral cell column (nucleus)
35	Parasympathetic ganglion neuron

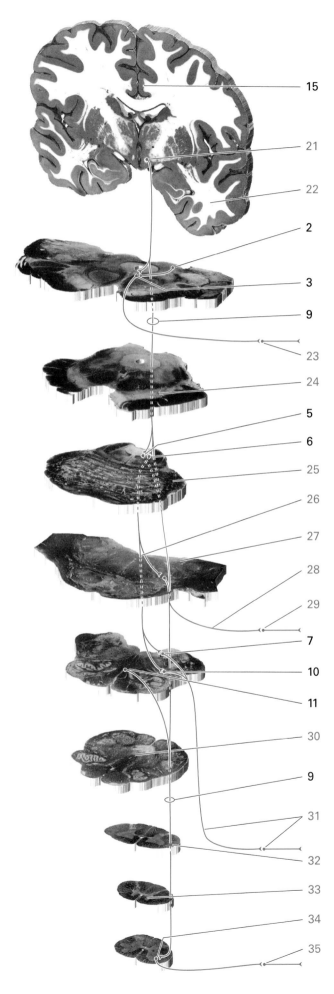

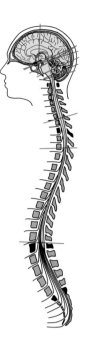

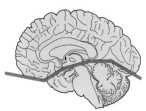

Visual Pathways

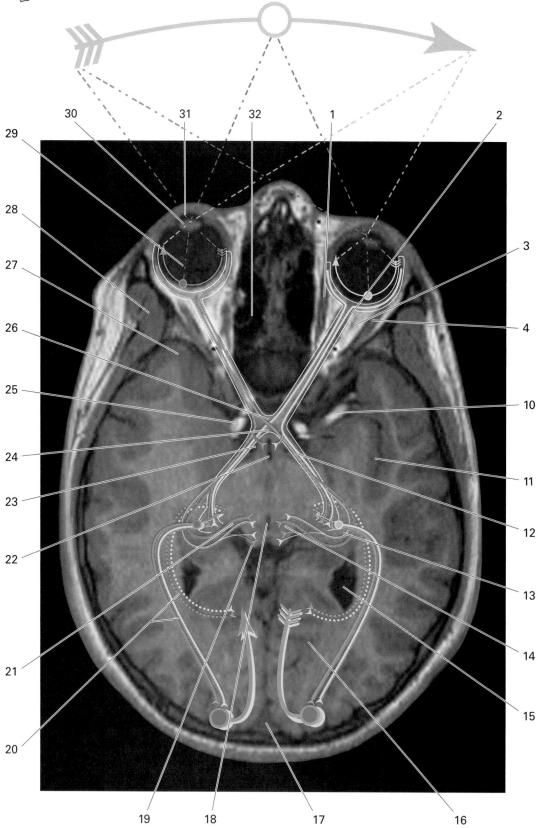

1 Medial rectus muscle
2 Optic nerve (CN II)
3 Orbital fat
4 Lateral rectus muscle
5 Corpus callosum
6 Fornix
7 Pituitary gland
8 Cerebral aqueduct (aqueduct of *Sylvius*)
9 Cerebellum
10 Middle cerebral artery, stem
11 Insula
12 Optic tract
13 Thalamus, dorsal lateral geniculate nucleus (dLGN) (lateral geniculate body)
14 Pretectal area
15 Lateral ventricle, trigone (atrium)
16 Calcarine (striate) cortex (*Brodmann*'s area 17)
17 Superior sagittal sinus
18 Cerebral aqueduct (aqueduct of *Sylvius*)
19 Superior colliculus
20 Optic radiation
21 Thalamus, medial geniculate nucleus (MG) (medial geniculate body)
22 Third ventricle (III)
23 Hypothalamus, suprachiasmatic nucleus
24 Infundibulum (pituitary stalk)
25 Internal carotid artery, supraclinoid part
26 Optic chiasm
27 Temporal pole
28 Temporalis muscle
29 Vitreous body of eye
30 Lens of eye
31 Cornea of eye
32 Ethmoidal air cells

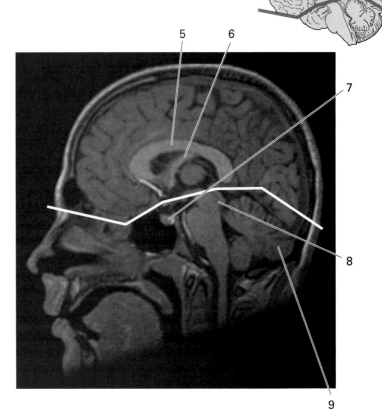

These pathways convey visual information for recognizing scenes and objects, directing gaze, controlling light levels on the retina, and modulating body function with changes in the length of the day.

[NB: The layout of the entire visual pathway is depicted here in an MRI assembled from different planes, as shown at the upper right.]

Light entering the **eyes** through the **cornea and lens** is inverted and focused on the **retina** to form an image. The arrow left to right in the visual fields has the center of gaze for the two eyes marked (circle). Sensory receptors transduce light, which is transferred to first-order neurons in the neural retina. These cells synapse on the second-order **retinal ganglion cells,** the axons of which leave the eye in the **optic (CN II) nerves.** After they enter the cranial cavity, the optic nerves join at the **optic chiasm,** where axons from the medial (nasal) retinae cross the midline. Each **optic tract** contains axons from the two eyes, which terminate in the **suprachi-asmatic nucleus** of the **hypothalamus** (to modulate circadian rhythms), the **superior colliculus** (to direct gaze), and the **pretectal area** (to control light levels through the pupils). The main termination is in the **thalamus** (especially the **dorsal lateral geniculate (dLGN) nucleus),** for form vision of the opposite visual field (i.e., arrowheads and circles of the right visual field in the left dLGN and circles and feathers in the right dLGN). Third-order axons from the dLGN course in the **optic radiations** of the **internal capsule,** first anterior and then lateral to the **trigone (atrium)** of the **lateral ventricle,** sweeping superior and inferior to the **occipital (posterior) horn** of the **lateral ventricle** to terminate in the **calcarine (striate) cortex** (*Brodmann*'s area 17) on the banks of the **calcarine fissure.** The center of gaze (circles) is at the occipital poles, and peripheral vision (arrowheads and feathers) is anterior in the **calcarine (striate) cortex.**

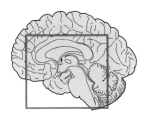

Olfactory Pathways

The sense of smell is used to distinguish a wide variety of odors, including what is commonly termed taste.

Approximately 30 small fiber bundles connect **olfactory receptor neurons** in the **olfactory epithelium** of the superior nasal cavity to the **olfactory bulbs.** The olfactory bulbs send axons to the **pyriform** and **entorhinal cortex (parahippocampal gyrus)** and the **cortical nucleus** of the **amygdala** in the **temporal lobe.** Direct connections are made also to the **anterior olfactory nucleus** and the **olfactory tubercle** of the **basal forebrain.** Second-order projections from all olfactory receiving areas in the temporal lobe are to the **dorsomedial nucleus (DM)** of the **thalamus** and the **lateral hypothalamic area** in the **diencephalon.** Olfactory areas of the temporal lobe also project to the **nucleus accumbens** and to the **insular** and **orbitofrontal cortex** (rendered schematically as they are not visible in this view of the brain) in the **telencephalon.** Fibers from the olfactory tubercle project to the **ventral pallidum** (a part of the substantia innominata) and from there to the dorsomedial nucleus (DM) of the thalamus and the lateral hypothalamic area. The anterior olfactory nucleus projects to the olfactory bulb and pyriform and entorhinal cortex (parahippocampal gyrus) of the opposite side.

1	Anterior commissure
2	Thalamus, dorsomedial nucleus (DM)
3	Hypothalamus, lateral area
4	Mamillary body
5	Amygdala
6	Prepyriform cortex
7	Olfactory tubercle and anterior olfactory nucleus
8	Lateral olfactory stria
9	Olfactory tract
10	Orbitofrontal cortex
11	Olfactory bulb
12	Cingulate gyrus
13	Medial olfactory stria
14	Nucleus accumbens

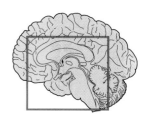

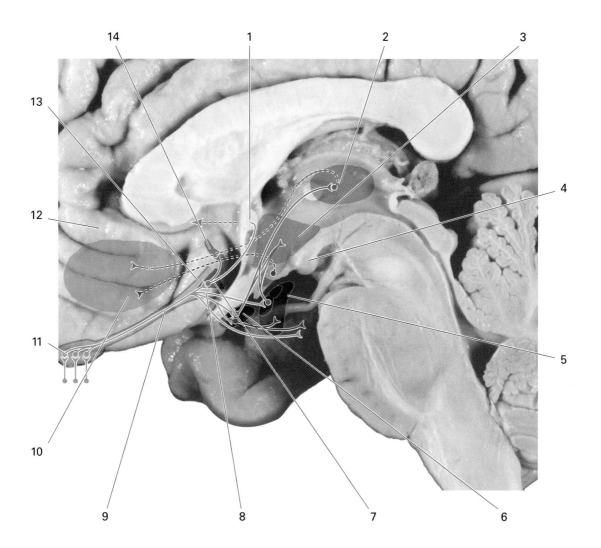

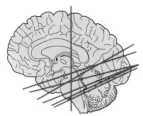

Auditory Pathways

Sound information for localization, discrimination, and speech is carried through a series of ipsilateral and contralateral pathways.

First-order axons from the **spiral ganglion** of the **cochlea** in the **acoustic part** of the **vestibulocochlear nerve (CN VIII)** synapse in the **dorsal** and **ventral cochlear nuclei**, next to the **inferior cerebellar peduncle (restiform body)** on the surface of the **brain stem** at the **pontomedullary junction**. **Second-order fibers** from the **dorsal cochlear nucleus** arch over the inferior cerebellar peduncle (restiform body) as the **dorsal acoustic stria** and pass medially in the dorsal **tegmentum** of the **pons** to the lateral aspect of the opposite tegmentum, where they ascend in the **lateral lemniscus**. Many fibers terminate in the lateral **superior olivary nucleus,** but the majority of lateral lemniscus fibers terminate in the **dorsal** and **ventral nuclei** of the **lateral lemniscus** and the **central nucleus** of the **inferior colliculus.**

Second-order fibers from the **ventral cochlear nucleus** reach the contralateral side as the **intermediate acoustic stria** by passing over the **inferior cerebellar peduncle (restiform body)** through the ipsilateral tegmentum to enter the **superior olivary nucleus**. Fibers cross the raphé and terminate in the opposite superior olivary nucleus. Some fibers enter the **lateral lemniscus** and terminate in the **nuclei** of the **lateral lemniscus** and the **inferior colliculus** of the opposite side.

Second-order fibers from the **ventral cochlear nucleus** take a third route, coursing under the **inferior cerebellar peduncle (restiform body)** and across the **ventral tegmentum** to form the **trapezoid body** that separates the tegmentum from the **pons, basilar part (basis pontis),** then cross the raphé and ascend in the contralateral **lateral lemniscus,** some fibers synapsing in the **superior olivary nucleus**. All fibers in the lateral lemniscus terminate in the **inferior colliculus.**

Third- and **higher-order fibers** from the **inferior colliculus** travel laterally in the **brachium** of the **inferior colliculus** to the **medial geniculate nucleus (MG)** of the **thalamus,** where they synapse. From the thalamus, **fourth-** and **higher-order axons** travel through the **internal capsule, sublenticular limb (acoustic radiation),** to the **transverse gyrus** (*Heschl's* **gyrus;** *Brodmann's* **areas 41** and **42**) on the **superior surface (superior temporal plane)** of the **temporal lobe.**

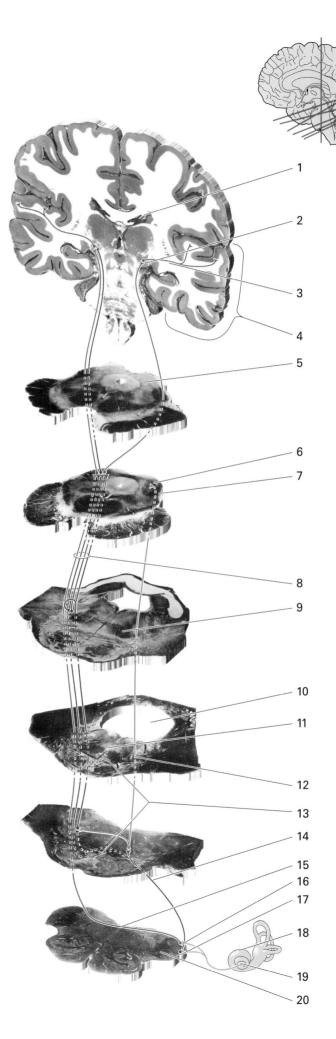

1 Lateral ventricle
2 Thalamus, medial geniculate nucleus (MG)
  (medial geniculate body)
3 Internal capsule, sublenticular limb (acoustic radiation)
4 Temporal lobe
5 Superior colliculus
6 Inferior colliculus
7 Inferior colliculus, brachium
8 Lateral lemniscus
9 Medial lemniscus
10 Fourth ventricle (IV)
11 Raphé
12 Superior olivary nucleus
13 Trapezoid body
14 Intermediate acoustic stria
15 Dorsal acoustic stria
16 Posterior (dorsal) cochlear nucleus (CN VIII)
17 Anterior (ventral) cochlear nucleus (CN VIII)
18 Cochlea
19 Spiral ganglion (CN VIII)
20 Inferior cerebellar peduncle (restiform body)

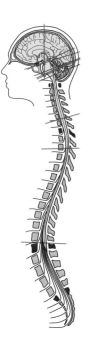

Vestibular Pathways

These pathways supply information from the vestibular apparatus about the position and movement of the head.

First-order fibers from the **vestibular ganglion** in the **vestibulocochlear nerve (CN VIII)** enter the **brain stem** at the **lateral pontomedullary junction** to synapse in four vestibular nuclei. These nuclei raise a visible eminence on the floor of the **fourth ventricle (IV)** from the **pons** to the medulla lateral to the **sulcus limitans** (pages 179, 180, and 184). The four **vestibular nuclei—superior, lateral, inferior,** and **medial**—give rise to vestibular pathways to the **cerebellum, spinal cord, brain stem**, and **thalamus**. First-order fibers also project directly to the **cerebellar vermian** and **floccular cortex** and the **fastigial nucleus.**

Second-order fibers from the **lateral vestibular nucleus** form the **lateral vestibulospinal tract,** which descends the length of the **spinal cord** in the ipsilateral **lateral funiculus** to terminate on motor and interneurons in the **anterior (ventral) horn.** Fibers from the **medial vestibular nuclei** descend in the **medial longitudinal fasciculus (MLF)** of the **anterior funiculus** on both sides to terminate in the medial **anterior (ventral) horn** of the **cervical spinal cord.**

Second-order vestibulocerebellar fibers arise mainly from the **inferior** and **medial vestibular nuclei** to enter the cerebellum via the **inferior cerebellar peduncle (restiform body),** through which the direct vestibulocerebellar fibers also travel, and terminate as **mossy fibers** in the **nodulus, uvula,** and **flocculus** of the **cerebellum.**

Second-order fibers from the **medial** and **superior vestibular nuclei** ascend in the **medial longitudinal fasciculus** of both sides to terminate in the cranial nerve **nuclei - abducent (CN VI), trochlear (CN IV),** and **oculomotor (CN III)** - of the extraocular muscles. Others ascend, mainly contralaterally after crossing in the **pons,** through the **lateral tegmentum** of the **pons** and **midbrain** to end in the **ventral posteromedial**

(VPM) and other **nuclei** of the **thalamus.** The thalamus projects through the **posterior limb** of the **internal capsule** to the lateral **parietal lobe** (*Brodmann*'s areas 2 and 3a).

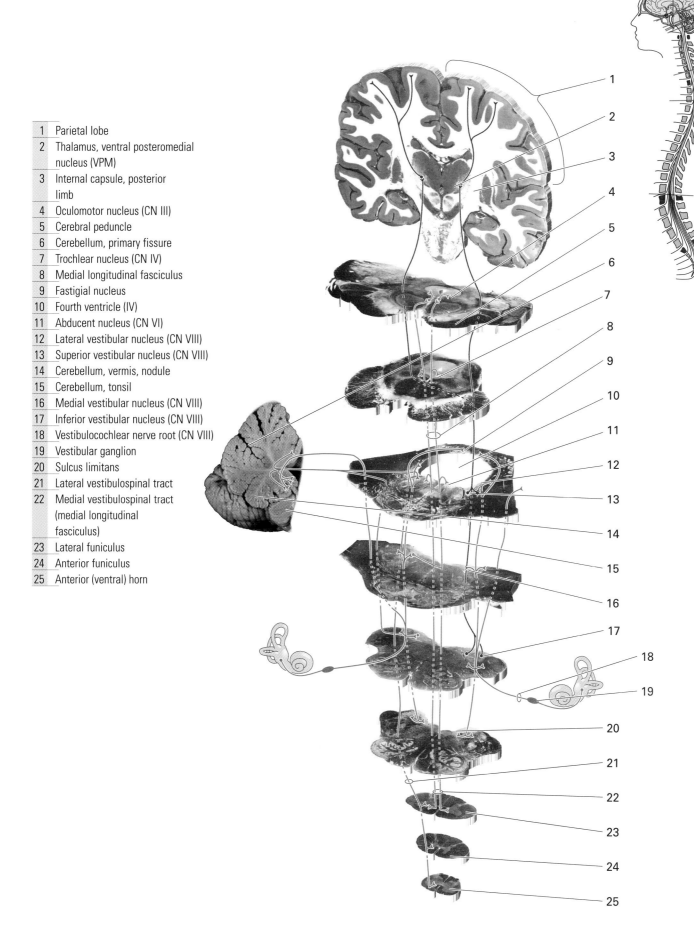

1   Parietal lobe
2   Thalamus, ventral posteromedial
    nucleus (VPM)
3   Internal capsule, posterior
    limb
4   Oculomotor nucleus (CN III)
5   Cerebral peduncle
6   Cerebellum, primary fissure
7   Trochlear nucleus (CN IV)
8   Medial longitudinal fasciculus
9   Fastigial nucleus
10 Fourth ventricle (IV)
11 Abducent nucleus (CN VI)
12 Lateral vestibular nucleus (CN VIII)
13 Superior vestibular nucleus (CN VIII)
14 Cerebellum, vermis, nodule
15 Cerebellum, tonsil
16 Medial vestibular nucleus (CN VIII)
17 Inferior vestibular nucleus (CN VIII)
18 Vestibulocochlear nerve root (CN VIII)
19 Vestibular ganglion
20 Sulcus limitans
21 Lateral vestibulospinal tract
22 Medial vestibulospinal tract
    (medial longitudinal
    fasciculus)
23 Lateral funiculus
24 Anterior funiculus
25 Anterior (ventral) horn

1
2
3
4
5
6
7
8
9
10
11
12
13
14
15
16
17
18
19
20
21
22
23
24
25

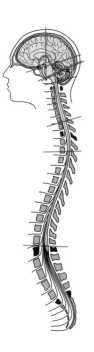

Corticospinal (Pyramidal) and Corticobulbar Pathways

This is the direct connection from the cerebral cortex for control of fine movements in the face and distal extremities, e.g., buttoning a jacket or playing a trumpet.

Axons from the **cerebral cortex** of the **precentral, prefrontal,** and **postcentral gyri** (*Brodmann's* **areas 4, 6, 8, 3, 2,** and **1**) course through the **corona radiata** to converge in the **posterior limb** of the **internal capsule.** They constitute the middle third of the **cerebral peduncle,** from which they enter the pons as the clustered fascicles of the **basilar** part of the **pons (basis pontis).** As the tract descends, a majority of fibers controlling fine movements of the face, mouth, jaw, tongue, pharynx, and larynx cross to motor nuclei of the **oculomotor (CN III), trochlear (CN IV), trigeminal (CN V), abducent (CN VI), facial (CN VII), glossopharyngeal (CN IX), vagal (CN X), accessory (CN XI),** and **hypoglossal nerves (CN XII)** (pages 183, 184, and 187). At the pontomedullary junction, the fibers emerge as the **pyramids (corticospinal tract)** on the anterior aspect of the **medulla oblongata.** In the caudal medulla, 65-90% of the fibers cross in the **pyramidal decussation (corticospinal tract)** to the opposite **lateral funiculus** of the **spinal cord** to become the **lateral corticospinal tract.** The remaining fibers descend in the ipsilateral **anterior funiculus** as the **anterior corticospinal tract.** Fibers are topographically arranged in the lateral
corticospinal tract: axons to cervical segments are medial to those to thoracic segments, which in turn are medial to fibers that end in the lumbar spinal cord. Axons of the lateral corticospinal tract terminate in the lateral **anterior (ventral) horn.** Axons in the anterior corticospinal tract cross in the **ventral white commissure** within a segment or two of termination in the opposite anterior horn. Corticospinal tract fibers form excitatory synapses on α motor neurons and interneurons of the **anterior (ventral) horn.**

1 Precentral, prefrontal, and postcentral
  gyri (*Brodmann's* areas 4, 6, 8, 3 a and b, 2, and 1)
2 Corona radiata
3 Red nucleus
4 Internal capsule, posterior limb
5 Trochlear nucleus (CN IV)
6 Inferior colliculus
7 Substantia nigra
8 Cerebral peduncle
9 Middle cerebellar peduncle (brachium pontis)
10 Pons, basilar part (basis pontis)
11 Nucleus ambiguus (ventral motor nucleus of
   vagus nerve) (CN X)
12 Cochlear nuclei (CN VIII)
13 Pyramids (corticospinal tracts)
14 Trigeminal (CN V) spinal nucleus
15 Pyramidal decussation (corticospinal tracts)
16 Lateral funiculus
17 Anterior (ventral) horn, lateral motor nuclei
18 Posterior (dorsal) horn
19 Anterior corticospinal tract
20 Posterior funiculus

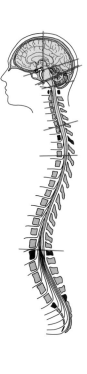

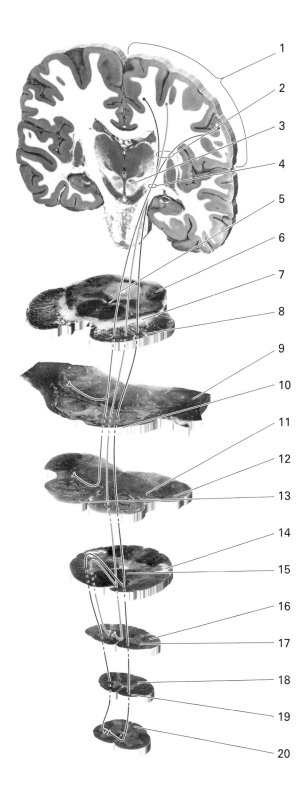

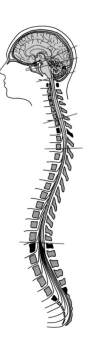

Rubrospinal and Tectospinal Pathways

The rubrospinal pathway (from the red nucleus) mediates voluntary control of movements, excepting the fine movements of the fingers, toes, and mouth. The tectospinal pathway (from the superior colliculus) mediates head and body orientation in response to localized visual, auditory, and tactile stimuli, often from the same source.

Rubrospinal fibers from the large cells of the caudal and medial **red nucleus** cross directly to the opposite side in the **anterior tegmental decussation** to descend in the lateral **pontine tegmentum** deep to the tract of the **trigeminal (CN V) spinal nucleus.** In the **medulla,** the rubrospinal fibers are adjacent to the **lateral reticular nucleus,** proceeding to the **lateral funiculus** of the **spinal cord,** where they are centered slightly anterior and medial to the **lateral corticospinal tract**, with whose fibers they are mixed. Rubrospinal fibers descend to midthoracic spinal segments. In the spinal cord, rubrospinal axons make excitatory synapses on interneurons between the **posterior (dorsal)** and **anterior (ventral) horns** and on a few motor neurons in the anterior (ventral) horn.

Tectospinal fibers arise from large cells in deeper layers of the **superior colliculus** and cross directly to the opposite side in the **posterior (dorsal) tegmental decussation.** Axons descend in the **pontine** and **medullary tegmentum** just ventral to the **medial longitudinal fasciculus** and into the **cervical spinal cord** in the **ventral funiculus** to terminate in the medial **anterior (ventral) horn** of the cervical spinal cord.

1	Posterior (dorsal) tegmental decussation (crossing of tectospinal tract)
2	Anterior tegmental decussation (crossing of rubrospinal tract)
3	Superior colliculus
4	Red nucleus
5	Thalamus, dorsal lateral geniculate nucleus (dLGN) (lateral geniculate body)
6	Pontine tegmentum
7	Superior cerebellar peduncle (brachium conjunctivum)
8	Medial lemniscus
9	Middle cerebellar peduncle (brachium pontis)
10	Inferior olive
11	Medial longitudinal fasciculus
12	Trigeminal (CN V) spinal nucleus
13	Lateral reticular nucleus
14	Pyramids (corticospinal tracts)
15	Lateral funiculus
16	Anterior (ventral) horn
17	Anterior funiculus
18	Posterior funiculus
19	Central canal
20	Anterior (ventral) median fissure (sulcus)

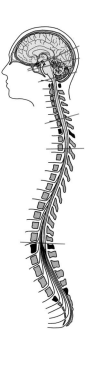

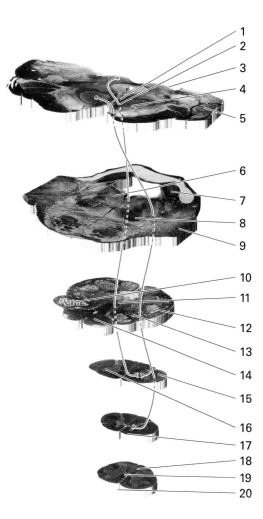

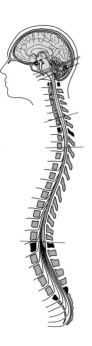

Reticulospinal Pathways

These tracts carry information from the brain stem reticular formation to the spinal cord to stabilize movement on uneven surfaces. Information to the spinal cord from the brain stem reticular formation is transmitted via this multisynaptic system from the reticular core of the medulla and pons.

The **medial (pontine) reticulospinal tract** arises from the **pontine reticular formation (oral and caudal parts)** in the **pontine tegmentum** and descends in the ipsilateral **medial longitudinal fasciculus** of the **brain stem** into the anterior and medial aspect of the **anterior funiculus** of the **spinal cord** to terminate on neurons in the **anterior (ventral) horn, medial motor nuclei.**

The **lateral (medullary) reticulospinal tract** arises in the **gigantocellular nucleus** of the dorsal **tegmentum** of the **medullary reticular formation.** Fibers of this tract descend, crossed and uncrossed, dorsal to the **inferior olivary nucleus** and lateral to the **dorsal accessory olivary nucleus.** In the **spinal cord** they course in the **lateral funiculus** ventral and lateral to the anterior horn. The tract terminates on neurons of the **anterior (ventral) horn, lateral motor nuclei.**

1	Pontine tegmentum
2	Fourth ventricle (IV)
3	Pontine reticular formation, oral part
4	Medial lemniscus
5	Pontine reticular formation, caudal part
6	Medial longitudinal fasciculus
7	Inferior cerebellar peduncle (restiform body)
8	Dorsal accessory olivary nucleus
9	Gigantocellular nucleus
10	Spinothalamic tracts (anterior and lateral)
11	Inferior olivary nucleus
12	Anterior (ventral) horn
13	Posterior funiculus
14	Lateral funiculus
15	Anterior funiculus

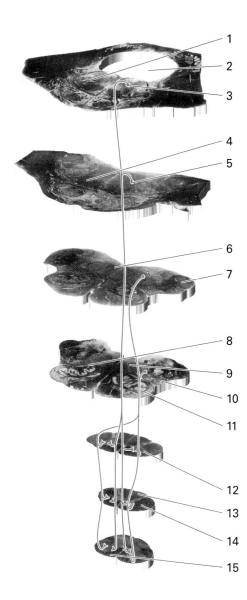

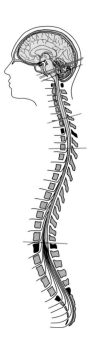

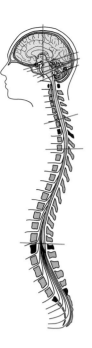

Cerebellar Pathways: Afferents

These tracts carry information to the cerebellum from the spinal cord, vestibular apparatus and nuclei, medulla, pons, reticular formation of the brain stem, and cerebral cortex. Axon collaterals of all the afferent cerebellar pathways end in the deep cerebellar nuclei.

Spinocerebellar Fibers

Spinocerebellar fibers (red) are carried in four tracts. **First-order** large myelinated **dorsal root axons** ascend from caudal segments in the **posterior (dorsal) columns** to upper lumbar and thoracic segments (T1 to L2) of the **spinal cord.** There they synapse on large neurons in the **dorsal (posterior) nucleus (*Clarke's* column),** which give rise to **second-order fibers** that form the **dorsal spinocerebellar tract.** These large axons carry information from the lower extremity and trunk in the ipsilateral **lateral funiculus** and enter the **cerebellum** via the **inferior cerebellar peduncle (restiform body)** to terminate as **mossy fibers** in the **vermian** and **paramedian cerebellar cortex** of the **posterior** and **anterior lobes.** Fibers from the superior dorsal roots, C2 to T1, ascend in the posterior columns and synapse in the **accessory (lateral) cuneate nucleus** of the same side. From there, **second-order cuneocerebellar axons** join those from the dorsal spinocerebellar tracts, reaching the cerebellum via the **inferior cerebellar peduncle (restiform body)** to terminate as **mossy fibers** in the **vermian and paramedian cerebellar cortex.**

First-order neurons in **dorsal roots** (L1 to S5) project to the **posterior (dorsal) horn** of the **spinal cord. Second-order axons** cross to the opposite side in the **ventral white commissure** to form the **anterior spinocerebellar tract** in the lumbar cord, which ascends in the **lateral funiculus.** At superior levels, axons from the ipsilateral dorsal horn (C2 to T1) form the **rostral spinocerebellar tract.** The anterior and rostral spinocerebellar tracts ascend in the **lateral tegmentum** of the **medulla** and **pons,** to enter the cerebellum via the **superior cerebellar peduncle (brachium conjunctivum).** Some of these fibers recross in the **cerebellar commissure;** all end as **mossy fibers** in the rostral and caudal **vermis.**

Reticulocerebellar Fibers

Reticulocerebellar fibers (green) arise from the ipsilateral **lateral reticular nucleus** in the lateral **medulla** dorsal to the **inferior olivary nucleus.** The axons course superficially over the lateral medulla and ascend in the **inferior cerebellar peduncle (restiform body)** to terminate in the cortex of the **vermis** as **mossy fibers.**

Vestibulocerebellar Fibers

Vestibulocerebellar fibers (not shown) arise from the ipsilateral vestibular apparatus and vestibular nuclei, reaching the cerebellar cortex via the **inferior cerebellar peduncle (restiform body)** and terminating as **mossy fibers** in the **cerebellar vermian** and **floccular cortex** and the **fastigial nucleus** (Vestibular Pathways, page 208).

Olivocerebellar Fibers

Olivocerebellar fibers (violet) originate from the **inferior olivary nuclei.** They leave the medial aspect of nucleus through the **hilum,** cross the midline, and enter the **inferior cerebellar peduncle (restiform body).** They terminate as **climbing fibers** in the **vermian, paramedian,** and **hemispheric cerebellar cortex.**

Corticopontocerebellar Fibers

Corticopontocerebellar fibers (blue) from most of the cerebral cortex join the **internal capsule** and descend in the **cerebral peduncles** to end in ipsilateral **pontine nuclei.** Axons from these cells cross in the pons to form the **middle cerebellar peduncle (brachium pontis)** and terminate as **mossy fibers** in the **cerebellar hemisphere.**

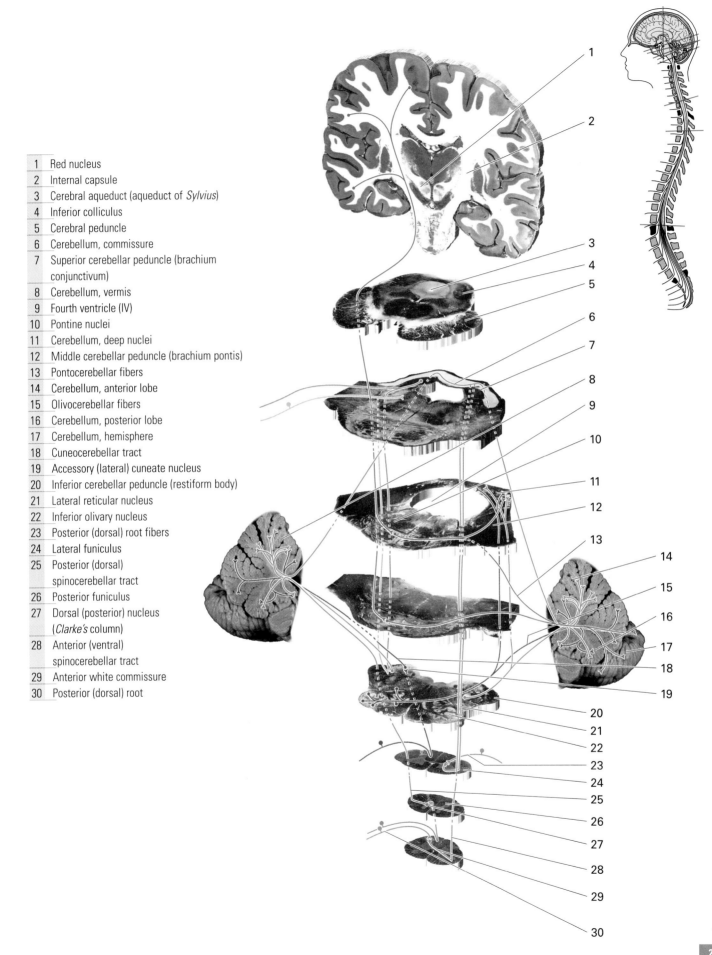

1 Red nucleus
2 Internal capsule
3 Cerebral aqueduct (aqueduct of *Sylvius*)
4 Inferior colliculus
5 Cerebral peduncle
6 Cerebellum, commissure
7 Superior cerebellar peduncle (brachium conjunctivum)
8 Cerebellum, vermis
9 Fourth ventricle (IV)
10 Pontine nuclei
11 Cerebellum, deep nuclei
12 Middle cerebellar peduncle (brachium pontis)
13 Pontocerebellar fibers
14 Cerebellum, anterior lobe
15 Olivocerebellar fibers
16 Cerebellum, posterior lobe
17 Cerebellum, hemisphere
18 Cuneocerebellar tract
19 Accessory (lateral) cuneate nucleus
20 Inferior cerebellar peduncle (restiform body)
21 Lateral reticular nucleus
22 Inferior olivary nucleus
23 Posterior (dorsal) root fibers
24 Lateral funiculus
25 Posterior (dorsal) spinocerebellar tract
26 Posterior funiculus
27 Dorsal (posterior) nucleus (*Clarke's* column)
28 Anterior (ventral) spinocerebellar tract
29 Anterior white commissure
30 Posterior (dorsal) root

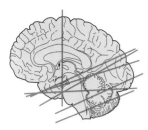

Cerebellar Pathways: Efferents

Efferent fibers from the cerebellum project to the brain stem and thalamus to modulate a variety of motor and other functions.

The output of the cerebellum arises from the **dentate, emboliform, globose,** and **fastigial nuclei** (the **deep cerebellar nuclei**), exiting mainly in the **superior cerebellar peduncle (brachium conjunctivum),** although some axons exit via the **inferior cerebellar peduncle (restiform body).**

The **dentate nucleus** (blue) projects the main output of the cerebellum through the **superior cerebellar peduncle,** decussating in the caudal **midbrain** at the level of the **inferior colliculus.** It synapses in or passes by the medial aspect of the **red nucleus** to end in the **ventral lateral (VL)** and **intralaminar nuclei** of the **thalamus,** which sends fibers to the **precentral gyrus** and **cerebral cortex** just rostral to it. Dentate nuclear fibers form a descending limb of the superior cerebellar peduncle and project to the opposite **pontine reticular formation** and to the **principal, medial accessory,** and **dorsal accessory olivary nuclei** of the **medulla.** The **emboliform** and **globose** (together the **interposed**) **nuclei** (red) project via the superior cerebellar peduncle to the opposite caudal **red nucleus** and to the **ventral posterior lateral (VPL)** and **intralaminar nuclei** of the **thalamus.** Fibers from the **fastigial nucleus** (brown) project to the ipsilateral and contralateral **vestibular nuclei (CN VIII)** via the **inferior** and **superior cerebellar peduncles.** Fastigial axons also terminate in the **ventral lateral (VL), ventral posterior lateral (VPL),** and **intralaminar nuclei** of the **thalamus.** The **vermian, flocculonodular,** and **uvular cerebellar cortex** (mustard) send fibers directly via the ipsilateral **inferior cerebellar peduncle (restiform body)** to the ipsilateral **vestibular nuclei (CN VIII).**

1   Thalamus, intralaminar nuclei
2   Thalamus, ventral lateral nucleus (VL)
3   Lateral sulcus (*Sylvian* fissure)
4   Posterior commissure
5   Red nucleus
6   Thalamus, dorsal lateral geniculate nucleus
    (dLGN) (lateral geniculate body)
7   Lateral lemniscus
8   Cerebral peduncle
9   Superior cerebellar peduncle (brachium conjunctivum)
10 Cerebellum, vermis
11 Fastigial nucleus
12 Dentate nucleus
13 Cerebellum, hemisphere
14 Cerebellum, flocculus
15 Pontine reticular formation
16 Inferior cerebellar peduncle (restiform body)
17 Medial accessory olivary nucleus
18 Dorsal accessory olivary nucleus
19 Principal olivary nucleus
20 Pyramids (corticospinal tracts)

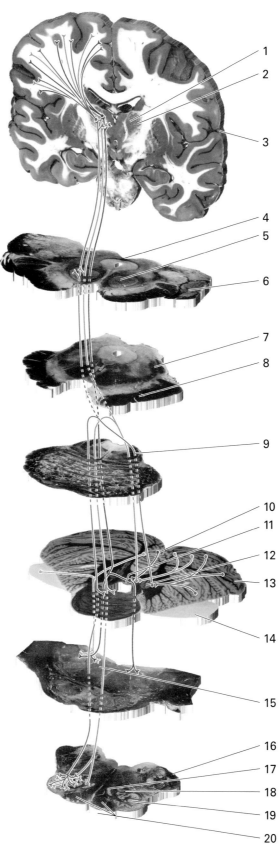

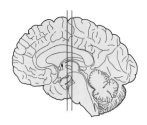

Basal Ganglia Pathways

The basal ganglia inhibit unwanted movement patterns and permit selected ones. They may also inhibit unwanted mental activities, such as inappropriate utterances, and permit selected ones, such as proper speech.

The basal ganglia are telencephalic and diencephalic nuclei, which include the **caudate nucleus** and **putamen** (together the **striatum**), the **globus pallidus**, the **subthalamic nucleus**, and the **substantia nigra**.

Wide areas of the **cerebral cortex** project topographically to the **caudate nucleus** and **putamen** and to the **subthalamic nucleus** and **substantia nigra** (blue). Fibers from the putamen and caudate nucleus project to the **globus pallidus, external (lateral)** and **internal (medial) segments (GPe and GPi)**, and **substantia nigra, pars reticulata (reticular part)**, through the **pallidoreticular (lenticulonigral) tract** (brown). The **substantia nigra, pars compacta (compact part)**, sends dopaminergic fibers back to the striatum via the **nigrostriatal tract** (red). The striatum also receives inputs from **intralaminar nuclei** of the **thalamus** (yellow). The **globus pallidus, external (lateral) segment (GPe)**, projects to and receives from the **subthalamic nucleus** (violet) via the **subthalamic fasciculus**, which penetrates the **internal capsule**. The **globus pallidus, external (lateral) segment (GPe)**, sends fibers medially via the **ansa lenticularis**, which course anteriorly around the internal capsule, where they are joined by fibers from substantia nigra, pars reticulata. The globus pallidus, internal (medial) segment (GPi), sends fibers that penetrate the internal capsule medially via the **lenticular fasciculus** (H2 field of *Forel*, mustard). Both bundles converge in the **subthalamus** (H field of *Forel*, which lies superior to the red nucleus), through which they pass before swinging superior and anterior in the **thalamic fasciculus** (H1 field of *Forel*, mustard) to terminate in the **ventral anterior (VA)** and **ventral lateral (VL) nuclei** of the **thalamus**.

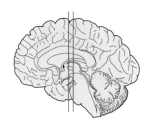

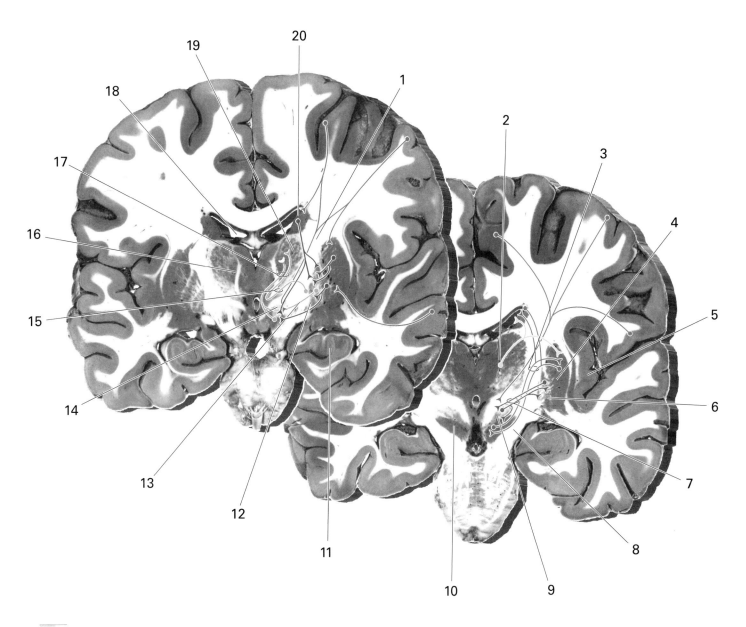

1	Internal capsule
2	Thalamus, intralaminar nuclei
3	Pallidoreticular (lenticulonigral) and nigrostriatal tracts
4	Putamen
5	Insula
6	Globus pallidus, external (lateral) segment (GPe)
7	Subthalamic fasciculus
8	Pyramid (corticospinal tract)
9	Subthalamic nucleus
10	Substantia nigra
11	Hippocampus
12	Globus pallidus, internal (medial) segment (GPi)
13	Ansa lenticularis
14	Subthalamus (H field of *Forel*)
15	Lenticular fasciculus (H2 field of *Forel*)
16	Mamillothalamic tract (fasciculus)
17	Thalamic fasciculus (H1 field of *Forel*)
18	Lateral ventricle
19	Thalamus, ventral anterior (VA) and ventral lateral (VL) nuclei
20	Caudate nucleus

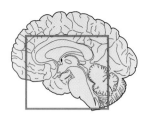

Hippocampal Pathways: Afferents

The hippocampus processes experience into memories and is involved in the recall of spatial locations.

Inputs from the "association cortex" in the **frontal lobe (*Brodmann*'s areas** [circled numbers] **12, 13, and 25), occipital lobe (area 19),** and **temporal lobe (areas 20, 22, and 38)** supply information from the senses by direct projections to the **entorhinal cortex (parahippocampal gyrus) (area 28)**. The entorhinal cortex projects across the **hippocampal fissure** via the "perforant" path to *Ammon*'s horn. Cortex in the **frontal lobe (areas 9 and 46)** and **parietal lobe (areas 7 and 23)** projects directly to *Ammon*'s **horn**. Fibers from the **amygdala (basal and lateral nuclei)** convey visceral information to the hippocampus via **area 28**. Axons from the **anterior** and **midline thalamic nuclei** travel through the **cingulum** to the **entorhinal cortex (parahippocampal gyrus)** or project directly to the hippocampus. Projections from the **basal forebrain (septum** and **diagonal band)** course through the **fornix,** with a smaller contingent traveling directly through the **stem** of the **temporal lobe** to end in **area 28** and the **hippocampus** proper. Projections from the **supramamillary region** of the **hypothalamus** course through the **fornix** to the **entorhinal cortex (parahippocampal gyrus)** and the hippocampus proper. In *Ammon*'s horn, information is processed through local hippocampal circuits from the **dentate gyrus** to *Ammon*'s **horn** to the **subiculum**.

1	Thalamus, anterior nucleus (A)
2	Fornix
3	Afferent cortical fibers from cingulate gyrus (*Brodmann*'s areas 23 and 24)
4	Thalamus, midline nuclei
5	Afferent cortical fibers from parietal cortex (*Brodmann*'s area 7)
6	Afferent cortical fibers from the superior temporal gyrus (*Brodmann*'s area 22)
7	Afferent cortical fibers from the occipital lobe (*Brodmann*'s area 19)
8	Subiculum
9	Dentate gyrus
10	Hypothalamus, supramamillary nucleus
11	Hippocampus, *Ammon*'s horn
12	Afferent cortical fibers via entorhinal cortex (parahippocampal gyrus) from inferior temporal gyrus (*Brodmann*'s area 20)
13	Entorhinal cortex (parahippocampal gyrus)
14	Amygdala, basal and lateral nuclei
15	Afferent cortical fibers via entorhinal cortex (parahippocampal gyrus) from temporal pole (*Brodmann*'s area 38)
16	Hippocampus, fimbria
17	Dentate gyrus
18	Parasubiculum
19	Entorhinal cortex (parahippocampal gyrus)
20	Presubiculum
21	Hippocampal sulcus
22	Subiculum
23	Hippocampus, CA3
24	Hippocampus, CA2
25	Hippocampus, CA1
26	Afferent cortical fibers via entorhinal cortex (parahippocampal gyrus) from gyrus rectus (straight gyrus) (*Brodmann*'s areas 12 and13)
27	Afferent cortical fibers via entorhinal cortex (parahippocampal gyrus) from preterminal gyrus (*Brodmann*'s area 25)
28	Nuclei of diagonal band (gyrus, band of *Broca*), horizontal and vertical limbs
29	Afferent cortical fibers via entorhinal cortex (parahippocampal gyrus) from insula
30	Septal nuclei
31	Anterior commissure
32	Fornix, precommissural fibers
33	Fornix, postcommissural fibers
34	Cingulum
35	Afferent cortical fibers from prefrontal cortex (*Brodmann*'s areas 46 and 9)

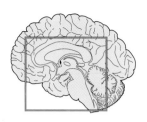

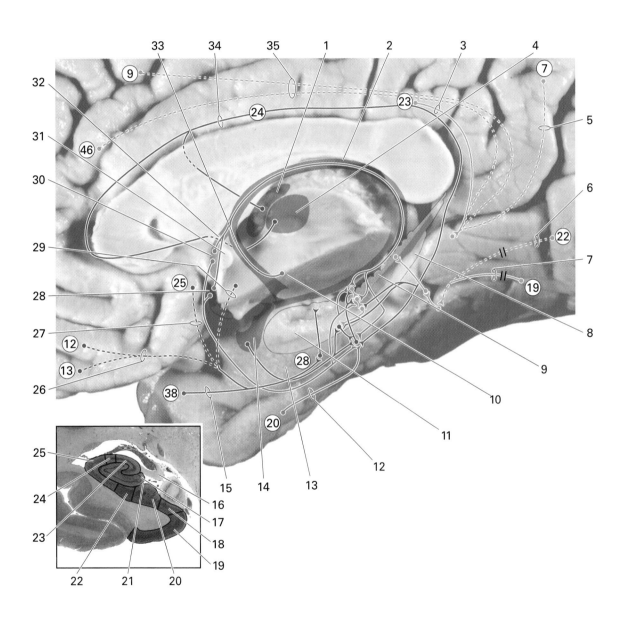

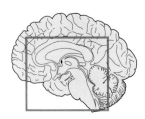

Hippocampal Pathways: Efferents

The hippocampus processes experience into memories and is involved in the recall of spatial locations.

Outputs of the hippocampus originate from *Ammon*'s **horn** and the **subiculum.** Fibers from the subiculum travel in the **fornix,** which is split by the **anterior commissure.** Fibers in the **precommissural fornix** end in the **septal nuclei, nucleus accumbens, preoptic nucleus** of the **hypothalamus,** and the **anterior olfactory nucleus** and project to the **medial frontal cortex** and **cortex** in the **gyrus rectus (straight gyrus)** including (***Brodmann*'s areas** [circled numbers] **11, 12, 13, 25** and **32).** Fibers of the **postcommissural fornix** end in the **interstitial nucleus** of the **stria terminalis, anterior nucleus (A)** of the **thalamus,** and **ventromedial** and **lateral mamillary nuclei** of the **hypothalamus.** Other fibers from the subiculum terminate directly in the **basal** and **lateral nuclei** of the **amygdala, entorhinal cortex (parahippocampal gyrus, area 28), retrosplenial cortex (areas 29** and **30),** and, via the **cingulum,** the **cingulate cortex (area 23).** Those from *Ammon*'s **horn** terminate in the **septal nuclei** via the **precommissural fornix.**

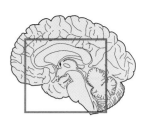

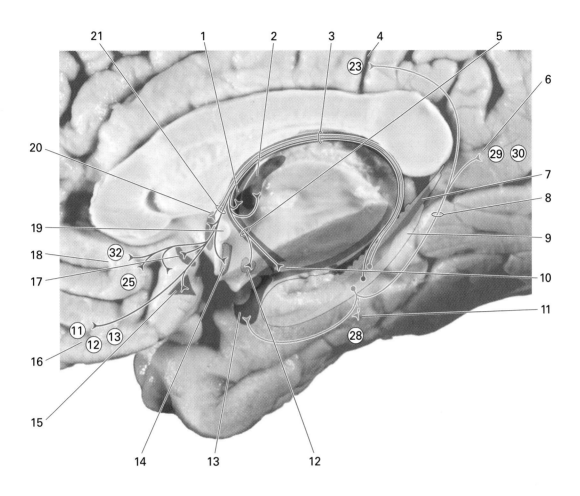

1	Stria terminalis, interstitial nucleus	12	Hypothalamus, ventromedial nucleus
2	Thalamus, anterior nucleus (A)	13	Amygdala, basal and lateral nuclei
3	Fornix	14	Hypothalamus, medial and lateral preoptic nuclei
4	Cingulate cortex (*Brodmann's* area 23)	15	Anterior olfactory nucleus
5	Fornix, postcommissural fibers	16	Gyrus rectus (straight gyrus)
6	Retrosplenial cortex (*Brodmann's* areas 29 and 30)		(*Brodmann's* areas 11, 12, and 13)
7	Hippocampus, *Ammon's* horn	17	Nucleus accumbens
8	Cingulum	18	Medial frontal cortex (*Brodmann's* areas 25 and 32)
9	Subiculum	19	Anterior commissure
10	Hypothalamus, lateral mamillary nucleus	20	Septal nuclei
11	Entorhinal cortex (parahippocampal gyrus) (*Brodmann's* area 28)	21	Fornix, precommissural fibers

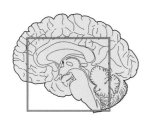

Amygdalar Pathways: Afferents

The amygdala integrates information from the senses and from within the body (visceral afferents) with past experience.

The **amygdala** ("almond") contains five nuclei in three groups: the **central nucleus**, the **cortical** and **medial nuclei**, and the **basal** and **lateral nuclei**. The amygdala receives connections from diverse regions of the **forebrain (telencephalon** and **diencephalon), midbrain,** and **brain stem.** These regions and amygdalar nuclei seen in cross section in the inset are projected on the mesial aspect of the brain.

There are five main pathways into the amygdala. From the **cerebral cortex,** axons from the **temporal lobe** connect to all amygdalar nuclei: the **insula** and *Brodmann's* **areas** (circled numbers) **22, 21, 20,** and **38** to the **central nucleus;** the **insula** and **areas 22, 21, 20, 38, 35,** and **36** and the **subiculum** to the **basal** and **lateral nuclei;** and the **subiculum** alone to the **cortical** and **medial nuclei.** Axons from *Brodmann's* **areas** (circled numbers) **12, 13, 14, 23, 24,** and **25** in the **frontal lobe** connect to the **central nucleus,** while those from **11, 12,** and **24** project to the **basal** and **lateral nuclei** (see inset). In the **stria terminalis** (the dorsal pathway), axons from the **interstitial nucleus** of the **stria terminalis** are joined by fibers from the **ventromedial nucleus** of the **hypothalamus** and **lateral hypothalamic area** to project to the **central, medial,** and **cortical nuclei** of the **amygdala.** The direct (ventral) pathway, ending also in the **central, medial,** and **cortical nuclei** of the **amygdala,** carries fibers through the stem of the **temporal lobe** from the **ventromedial nucleus** of the **hypothalamus,** lateral hypothalamic area, the **substantia innominata,** and the **nucleus** of the **diagonal band (gyrus, band of *Broca*). Fibers** from the **olfactory bulb** coursing though the **lateral olfactory stria** end directly in the **medial** and **cortical amygdalar nuclei;** in the **prepyriform cortex,** which then projects to the **lateral** and **basal amygdalar nuclei;** or in the **entorhinal cortex (parahippocampal gyrus) (area 28),** which then projects

to the **lateral** and **basal nuclei.** Diverse inputs reach all amygdalar nuclei through the **medial forebrain bundle:** fibers originate from the **median, parafascicular,** and **medial geniculate nuclei** of the **thalamus;** from the **ventral tegmental area, central mesencephalic gray, dorsal raphé nucleus, substantia nigra,** and the **peripeduncular nucleus** in the **midbrain;** and from the **lateral parabrachial nucleus, locus ceruleus,** and **solitary nucleus** in the **pons** and the **medulla.**

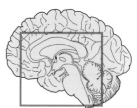

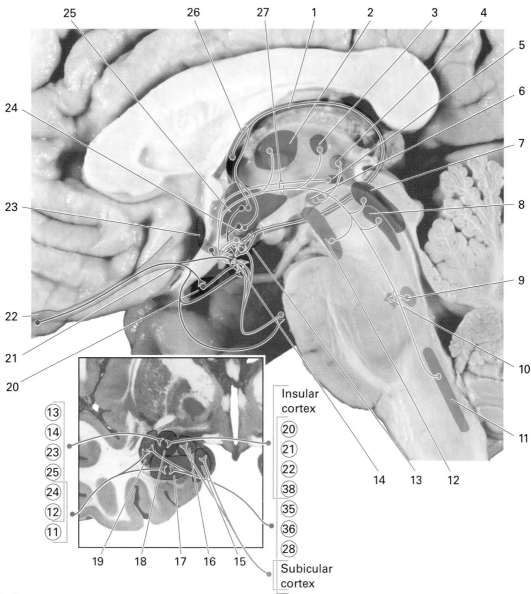

Insular
cortex

Subicular
cortex

1	Stria terminalis
2	Thalamus, median nuclei
3	Parafascicular nucleus
4	Thalamus, medial geniculate nucleus (MG) (medial geniculate body)
5	Peripeduncular nucleus
6	Ventral tegmental area
7	Periaqueductal (central) gray substance
8	Posterior (dorsal) raphé nucleus
9	Lateral parabrachial nucleus
10	Locus ceruleus
11	Solitary nucleus
12	Substantia nigra, pars compacta (compact part)
13	Amygdala, central nucleus
14	Amygdala, cortical and medial nuclei

15	Amygdala, cortical nucleus
16	Amygdala, medial nucleus
17	Amygdala, basal nucleus
18	Amygdala, central nucleus
19	Amygdala, lateral nucleus
20	Substantia innominata
21	Lateral olfactory stria
22	Olfactory bulb
23	Nucleus of diagonal band (gyrus, band of *Broca*), horizontal limb
24	Hypothalamus, ventromedial nucleus
25	Lateral hypothalamic area
26	Stria terminalis, interstitial nucleus
27	Medial forebrain bundle

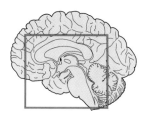

Amygdalar Pathways: Efferents

The amygdala integrates information from the senses and from within the body (visceral afferents) with past experience.

The five nuclei of the **amygdala**: the **central nucleus**, the **cortical** and **medial nuclei**, and the **basal** and **lateral nuclei** project widely throughout the **forebrain (telencephalon** and **diencephalon), midbrain**, and **brain stem**. The amygdalar nuclei seen in cross section in the inset are projected onto the midsagittal aspect of the brain.

Four groups of axons leave the **amygdala**. Forebrain targets of the **central nucleus** of the **amygdala** are the **substantia innominata, nuclei** of the **horizontal** and **vertical limbs** of the **diagonal band (gyrus, band of *Broca*)**, the **lateral hypothalamic area**, the **interstitial nucleus** of the **stria terminalis** and the **septal nuclei.** Axons from the **central nucleus** also course in the **medial forebrain bundle** to targets in the brain stem. In the **midbrain**, these end in the **parafascicular nucleus; ventral tegmental area; substantia nigra, pars compacta (compact part); peripeduncular nucleus; central mesencephalic gray;** and **the posterior (dorsal) raphé nucleus;** in the **pons** and **medulla,** they end in the **superior central nucleus; lateral parabrachial nucleus; locus ceruleus; nucleus subceruleus; raphé nuclei magnus, pallidus, and obscurus; nucleus** of the **solitary tract;** and the **dorsal nucleus** of the **vagus nerve.** Outputs of the **basal, lateral, medial,** and **cortical nuclei** travel in the **stria terminalis** to innervate the **interstitial nucleus** of the **stria terminalis;** and the **paraventricular, anterior, ventromedial,** and **preoptic nuclei** of the **hypothalamus.** Axons from the **basal** and **lateral amygdaloid nuclei** coursing through the **stria terminalis** also innervate the **caudate nucleus** and **putamen;** the **nucleus accumbens;** and the **olfactory tubercle** of the telencephalon. From the **basal** and **lateral nuclei,** some axons travel directly through the **stem** of the **temporal lobe** to the **septal nuclei** and the **nucleus** of the **vertical limb** of the **diagonal band (band of**

Broca). Cortical projections of **basal** and **lateral** nuclei are to the **frontal lobe (*Brodmann*'s areas** [circled numbers] **4, 6, 9, 10, 12, 13, 14, 25,** and **32),** the **temporal lobe (areas 35** and **36),** and the **insula.** The nearby **periamygdaloid cortex** projects to the **median nuclei** of the **thalamus** and the **lateral hypothalamic area.**

1	Stria terminalis
2	Thalamus, median nuclei
3	Parafascicular nucleus
4	Peripeduncular nucleus
5	Ventral tegmental area
6	Periaqueductal (central) gray substance
7	Posterior (dorsal) raphé nucleus
8	Superior central nucleus
9	Lateral parabrachial nucleus
10	Locus ceruleus
11	Nucleus subceruleus
12	Solitary nucleus
13	Dorsal (posterior) nucleus of vagus nerve (CN X)
14	Raphé nuclei, magnus, obscurus, and pallidus
15	Substantia nigra, pars compacta (compact part)
16	Amygdala, central nucleus
17	Amygdala, basal and lateral nuclei
18	Amygdala, cortical nucleus
19	Amygdala, medial nucleus
20	Amygdala, basal nucleus
21	Amygdala, central nucleus
22	Amygdala, lateral nucleus
23	Substantia innominata
24	Periamygdaloid cortex
25	Amygdala, cortical and medial nuclei
26	Olfactory tubercle
27	Nuclei of diagonal band (gyrus, band of *Broca*), horizontal and vertical limbs
28	Nucleus accumbens
29	Hypothalamus, medial preoptic nucleus
30	Hypothalamus, ventromedial nucleus
31	Caudate nucleus
32	Putamen
33	Septal nuclei
34	Hypothalamus, anterior nucleus
35	Hypothalamus, paraventricular nucleus
36	Stria terminalis, interstitial nucleus
37	Medial forebrain bundle

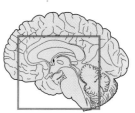

33 34 35 36 37 1 2 3

32

31

30

29

28

27

26

25

24

23

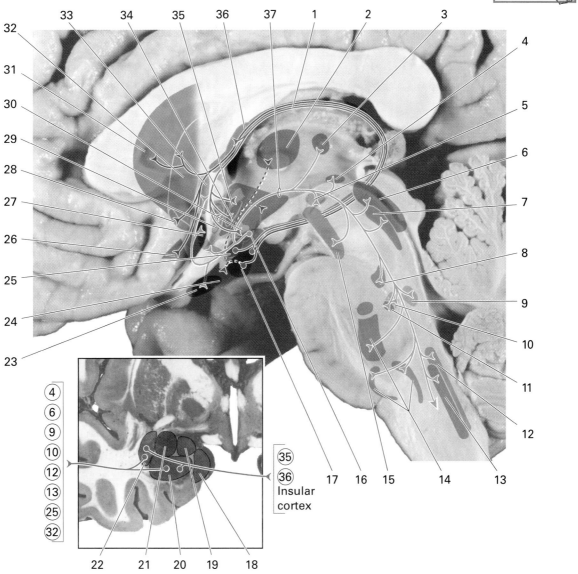

4
5
6
7
8
9
10
11
12
13

4
6
9
10
12
13
25
32

35
36
Insular
cortex

22 21 20 19 18

17 16 15 14 13

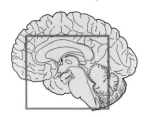

Hypothalamic Pathways: Afferents

The hypothalamus integrates external and internal stimuli to regulate the internal body environment, behaviors such as sleep and wakefulness, feeding, and sexual activity and to coordinate generalized responses through somatic motor activity, visceral control, and hormone release.

The **hypothalamus** consists of gray matter nuclei surrounding the anterior end of the **third ventricle (III)**. These nuclei can be grouped at three **levels** from front to back: chiasmatic, tuberal, and posterior. They also can be grouped in three medial to lateral **zones**. The periventricular and medial zones contain nuclei that are medial to the **lateral hypothalamic area** (the lateral zone), which consists of axons and dendrites (see inset). At the **chiasmatic level** are the **suprachiasmatic, paraventricular, anterior, supraoptic,** and **lateral** and **medial preoptic nuclei**. At the **tuberal level** are the **dorsomedial, ventromedial, arcuate,** and **tuberal nuclei**. At the **posterior level** are the **medial** and **lateral mamillary** and **posterior nuclei**. The **medial zone** contains all nuclei except the **paraventricular** and **arcuate nuclei**, which are the identified structures in the **periventricular zone**.

Afferents come from the **brain stem** (via the **dorsal longitudinal fasciculus, medial forebrain bundle,** and **mamillary peduncle**), the **thalamus** (via the **inferior thalamic peduncle**, not shown), the **hippocampus** (via the **fornix**), **amygdala** (via the **stria terminalis**), and **cerebral cortex** (via the **medial forebrain bundle**) and directly from the **olfactory bulb** and **eyes**. Inputs to the hypothalamus from below travel in three separate pathways: the **dorsal longitudinal fasciculus** from the **periaqueductal gray** in the **midbrain, pons,** and **medulla**; the **medial forebrain bundle** from the **midbrain** and **pontine tegmentum**, including the **parabrachial nuclei**; and the **mamillary peduncle** from the midbrain **tegmentum** and central gray. Information from the **thalamus** is conveyed in the **inferior thalamic peduncle** while the **fornix** carries inputs from the **hippocampus** to the **mamillary body**. The **medial forebrain**

bundle is the conduit for connections from the **frontal lobe, olfactory cortex, septum,** and **caudate nucleus**. Direct inputs from the **eye** to the **suprachiasmatic nucleus** are from the **optic tract**. Receptors in the hypothalamus sense temperature, glucose, hormones, pH, and pyrogens.

1	Stria terminalis
2	Mamillary peduncle
3	Medial forebrain bundle
4	Posterior (dorsal) longitudinal fasciculus
5	Periaqueductal and periventricular gray
6	Midbrain tegmentum
7	Hippocampus
8	Parabrachial nuclei
9	Solitary nucleus
10	Pontine tegmentum
11	Pons
12	Mamillothalamic tract
13	Hypothalamic sulcus
14	Hypothalmus, lateral area
15	Mamillary body (hypothalamus, medial and lateral mamillary nuclei)
16	Hypothalamus, posterior nucleus
17	Hypothalamus, tuberal nuclei
18	Hypothalamus, dorsomedial nucleus
19	Hypothalamus, ventromedial nucleus
20	Hypothalamus, arcuate (infundibular) nucleus
21	Hypothalamus, supraoptic nuclei
22	Hypothalamus, suprachiasmatic nucleus
23	Hypothalamus, lateral preoptic nucleus
24	Hypothalamus, anterior nucleus
25	Hypothalamus, medial preoptic nucleus
26	Hypothalamus, paraventricular nucleus
27	Fornix
28	Entorhinal cortex (parahippocampal gyrus)
29	Pituitary gland, anterior lobe
30	Pituitary gland, posterior lobe
31	Retinohypothalamic fibers
32	Amygdala
33	Septal nuclei
34	Corpus callosum
35	Caudate nucleus
36	Medial forebrain bundle
37	Interthalamic adhesion (massa intermedia)
38	Fornix

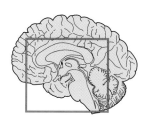

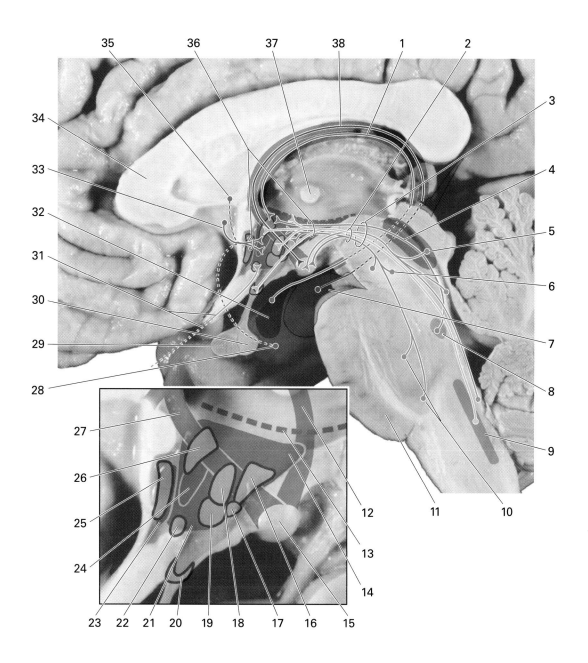

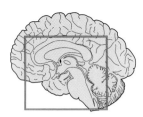

Hypothalamic Pathways: Efferents

The hypothalamus integrates external and internal stimuli to regulate the internal body environment, behaviors such as sleep and wakefulness, feeding, and sexual activity and to coordinate generalized responses through somatic motor activity, visceral control, and hormone release.

In spite of its small size, the hypothalamus projects widely throughout the brain. Descending pathways are through the **hypothalamospinal tract** to **brain stem** and **spinal cord** and the **dorsal longitudinal fasciculus** to brain stem to neurons which target **preganglionic** cells of the **autonomic nervous system**. The **mamillary bodies** project to the **dorsal tegmental nucleus** via the **mamillotegmental tract** and to the **anterior nucleus** of the **thalamus** through the **mamillothalamic tract**. Both of these tracts take origin from the stout **mamillary peduncle**. The **lateral preoptic nucleus** projects to **dorsomedial nucleus** of the **thalamus** through the **inferior thalamic peduncle** and the **lateral habenular nucleus** through the **stria medullaris**. The **preoptic region** sends fibers through the **stria terminalis** to the **central, cortical,** and **medial nuclei** of the **amygdala**. The **ventromedial hypothalamic nucleus** projects through the **medial forebrain bundle** to the **septal nuclei**. Cells in the **tuberal** and the **posterior hypothalamic nuclei** project to the entire **cortical mantle** of the same side (not shown). **Supraoptic** and **paraventricular (magnocellular) hypothalamic nuclei** send axons into the **posterior pituitary** to terminate on blood vessels where they release the hormones **oxytocin** and **vasopressin**. Neurons in the **periventricular** and **paraventricular nuclei** project to the **median eminence**. There they release peptide hormones – releasing factors – into the blood of the **hypophysial portal system** that effect secretion of hormones from the **anterior pituitary**.

1	Fornix
2	Stria terminalis
3	Mamillary peduncle
4	Medial forebrain bundle
5	Corpus callosum, splenium
6	Habenula, lateral nucleus
7	Pineal gland
8	Inferior colliculus
9	Mamillotegemental tract
10	Posterior (dorsal) longitudinal fasciculus
11	Fourth ventricle (IV)
12	Hypothalamospinal tract
13	Mamillary body (hypothalamus, medial and lateral mamillary nuclei)
14	Hypothalamus, posterior nucleus
15	Hypothalamus, tuberal nuclei
16	Oculomotor nerve (CN III)
17	Amygdala
18	Pituitary gland, posterior lobe
19	Optic chiasm
20	Hypothalamus, supraoptic nuclei
21	Hypothalamus, lateral preoptic nucleus
22	Anterior commissure
23	Hypothalamus, paraventricular nucleus
24	Mamillothalamic tract
25	Thalamus, anterior nucleus (A)
26	Stria medullaris of thalamus
27	Thalamus, dorsomedial nucleus (DM)

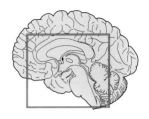

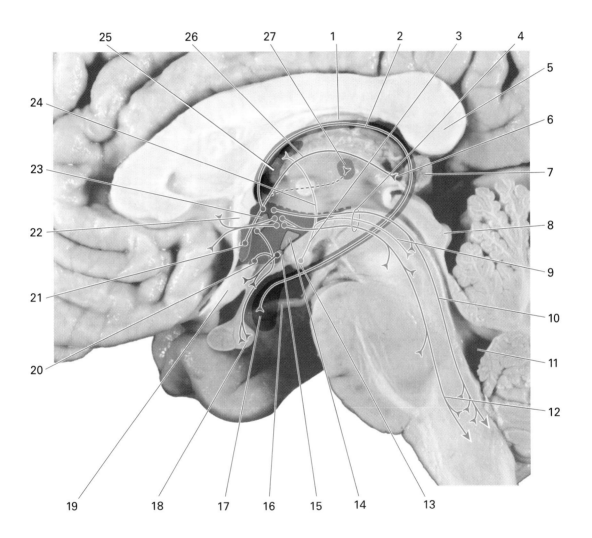

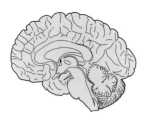

Cholinergic and Dopaminergic Pathways

Small numbers of neurons in the basal forebrain and brain stem that make dopamine and acetylcholine generally influence arousal, attention, mood, and cerebral blood flow. Disturbances of these systems are associated with Parkinson's disease, dystonia, and Alzheimer's disease.

Cholinergic neurons (red) in the **nucleus basalis (nucleus basalis** of **Meynert)** project widely through the **cingulum** to the medial **cerebral cortex,** through the **external** and **extreme capsules** to the **lateral cortex,** and through the **temporal stem** and **stria terminalis** to the **amygdala** and **temporal cortex.** Neurons in the **septal nuclei** connect through the **fornix** to the **hippocampus,** and cells in the **dorsal tegmental area** of the **pons** project to the **thalamus.**

Dopaminergic neurons (green) in the **substantia nigra, pars compacta (compact part),** project to the **striatum (caudate nucleus** and **putamen)** (see page 221), while those in the **ventral tegmental area** project superiorly via the **medial forebrain bundle** to the **septum** and **amygdala** and widely to the **cerebral cortex** (especially the **frontal lobe)** via the **cingulum.**

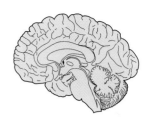

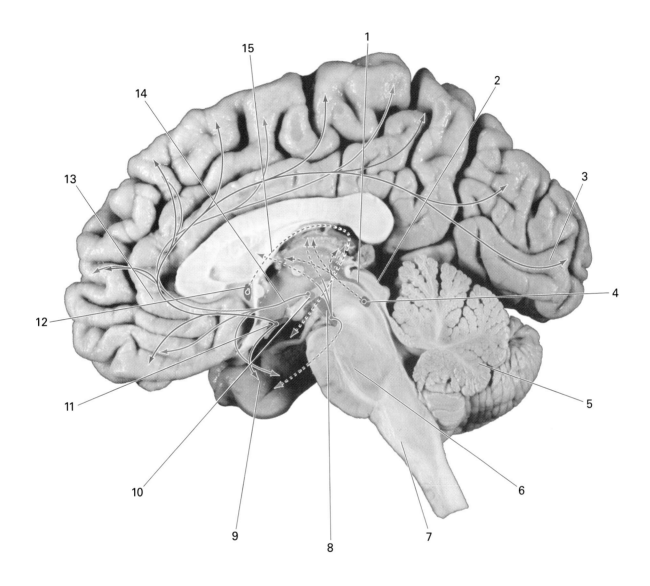

1	Cerebral aqueduct (aqueduct of *Sylvius*)
2	Superior and inferior colliculi (quadrigeminal plate, tectum)
3	Occipital lobe
4	Dorsal tegmental area
5	Cerebellum
6	Pons
7	Medulla
8	Substantia nigra, pars compacta (compact part)
9	Uncus
10	Ventral tegmental area
11	Nucleus basalis (nucleus basalis of *Meynert*)
12	Septal nuclei
13	Cingulate gyrus
14	Medial forebrain bundle
15	Fornix, column

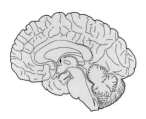

Noradrenergic and Serotonergic Pathways

Small numbers of neurons in the basal brain stem that make norepinephrine and serotonin strongly and generally influence arousal, attention, mood, and cerebral blood flow. Disturbances of these systems are associated with sleep disorders, depression, obsessive compulsive disorder, schizophrenia, substance abuse, and migraine headaches.

Noradrenergic neurons (mustard) in the **locus ceruleus** innervate the entire brain. This nucleus supplies the **brain stem** directly. It gives rise to a posterior midline pathway—the **dorsal noradrenergic bundle**—from which groups of fibers leave to supply the **cerebellum** through the **superior cerebellar peduncle** and the **thalamus** through the **internal** and **external medullary laminae.** The main bundle continues forward to join the **medial forebrain bundle** to supply the **hypothalamus.** Anteriorly, in the **basal forebrain**, fibers supply the **nucleus basalis (nucleus basalis** of *Meynert*) directly, the **hippocampus** via the **fornix,** and the **amygdala** and **temporal lobe** through the **temporal stem** and **stria terminalis.** The **cerebral cortex** throughout the hemispheres is supplied from the basal forebrain via **lateral** fibers through the **external** and **extreme capsules** and a **medial** route over the **corpus callosum** via the **lateral longitudinal striae** (of *Lancisi*) and the **cingulum.** Noradrenergic neurons in the nearby **nucleus subceruleus** innervate the **pons, medulla,** and, via the **lateral funiculus,** the **spinal cord.**

Serotonergic neurons (blue) are found in the midline **raphé nuclei** throughout the brain stem. Fibers project superiorly from the **posterior (dorsal) raphé nucleus** via the **medial forebrain bundle** to the **diencephalon,** the **basal ganglia,** and the **basal forebrain.** From the basal forebrain they distribute widely to the **cerebral cortex.** Diffuse projections to the **cerebellar cortex** from the **raphé nucleus obscurus** enter through the cerebellar peduncles. Spinal projections from the **nuclei raphé magnus, obscurus,** and **pallidus** are through the **lateral funiculus.**

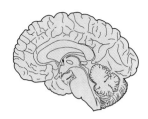

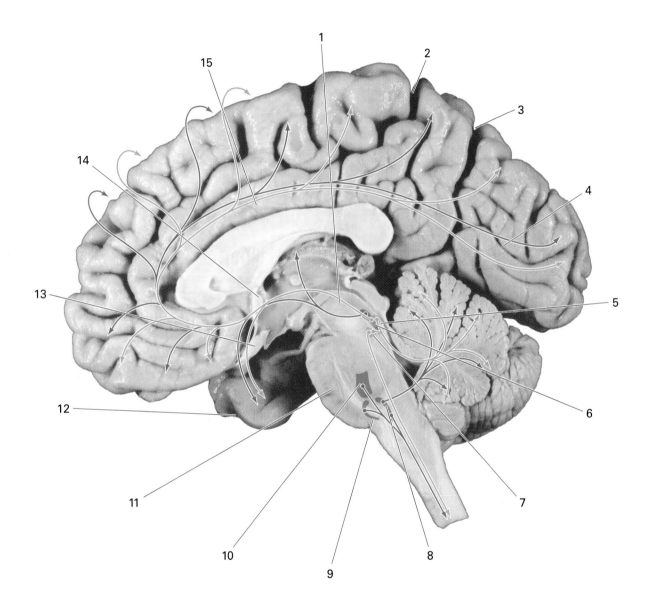

1   Midbrain tegmentum
2   Central sulcus (fissure of *Rolando*)
3   Parieto-occipital sulcus
4   Calcarine fissure
5   Pontine tegmentum
6   Locus ceruleus
7   Nucleus subceruleus
8   Raphé nucleus obscurus

9   Raphé nucleus pallidus
10 Raphé nucleus magnus
11 Pons
12 Temporal pole
13 Optic chiasm
14 Anterior commissure
15 Cingulate gyrus

Index

About the authors:

Joseph Hanaway, MD has more than 25 years experience as a practicing neurologist and has taught basic and clinical Neuroanatomy at Harvard University, the University of Virginia, Washington University, and the University of Missouri Schools of Medicine.

Thomas A. Woolsey, MD is a world renowned neurobiologist best known for his discovery of the cortical barrels in rodents. Since his appointment at Washington University School of Medicine 25 years ago, he has won numerous awards for his teaching to medical students, residents, and undergraduates in Psychology and the Life Sciences.

Mokhtar H. Gado, MD is an internationally known neuroradiologist with over 30 years of clinical and teaching experience at Washington University School of Medicine and the Mallinckrodt Institute of Radiology. Dr. Gado prepared the MRIs used throughout this book.

Melville P. Roberts, Jr., MD is the William Beecher Scoville Professor of Neurosurgery at the University of Connecticut School of Medicine. He has taught Neuroanatomy to medical students and practiced neurosurgery for over 30 years.

About the book:

Production Management: Susan Graham
Production Services: J/B Woolsey Associates and Thomas A. Woolsey
Interior Design: Ox and Company; J/B Woolsey Associates
and Thomas A. Woolsey
Illustration Development and Illustrations: J/B Woolsey Associates
Cover Design: Susan Brown Schmidler from an MRI by Mokhtar H. Gado
and Thomas A. Woolsey
Copyeditor: Sara Jenkins
Index: Craig Brown
Printer: Courier